Acupressure & Reflexology For Dummies

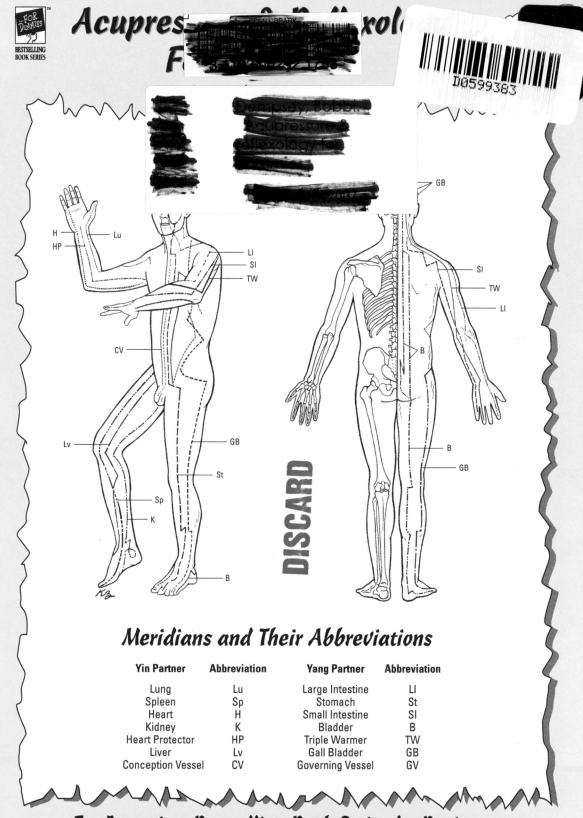

DISCARD

Meridians and Their Abbreviations

Yin Partner	Abbreviation	Yang Partner	Abbreviation
Lung	Lu	Large Intestine	LI
Spleen	Sp	Stomach	St
Heart	H	Small Intestine	SI
Kidney	K	Bladder	B
Heart Protector	HP	Triple Warmer	TW
Liver	Lv	Gall Bladder	GB
Conception Vessel	CV	Governing Vessel	GV

For Dummies: Bestselling Book Series for Beginners

Foot Reflexology Map

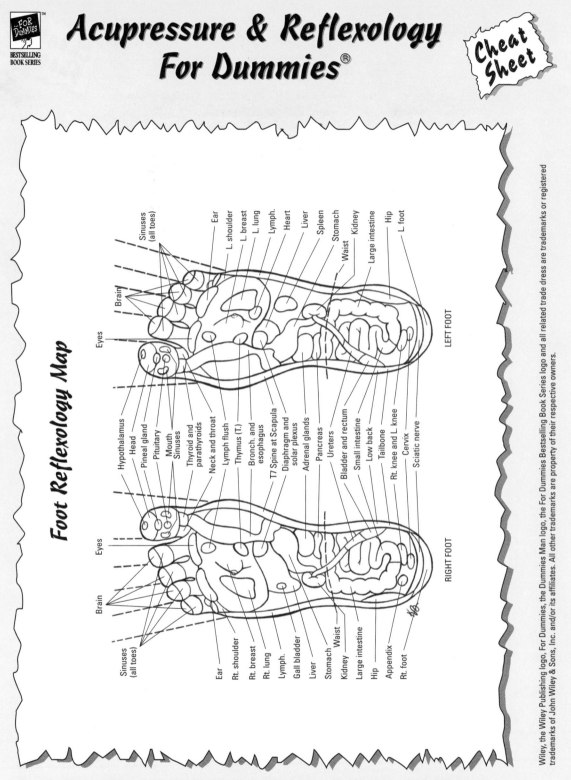

Labels (left foot): Sinuses (all toes), Ear, L. shoulder, L. breast, L. lung, Lymph., Heart, Liver, Spleen, Stomach, Kidney, Waist, Large intestine, Hip, L. foot, Brain, Eyes

LEFT FOOT

Labels (right foot): Hypothalamus, Head, Pineal gland, Pituitary, Mouth, Sinuses, Thyroid and parathyroids, Neck and throat, Lymph flush, Thymus (T.), Bronch. and esophagus, T7 Spine at Scapula, Diaphragm and solar plexus, Adrenal glands, Pancreas, Ureters, Bladder and rectum, Small intestine, Low back, Tailbone, Rt. knee and L. knee, Cervix, Sciatic nerve

Eyes, Brain

Sinuses (all toes), Ear, Rt. shoulder, Rt. breast, Rt. lung, Lymph., Gall bladder, Liver, Stomach, Waist, Kidney, Large intestine, Hip, Appendix, Rt. foot

RIGHT FOOT

For Dummies: Bestselling Book Series for Beginners

Acupressure & Reflexology

FOR

DUMMIES®

About the Authors

Synthia Andrews has been a massage and bodywork therapist for 25 years. She is an authorized teacher of Jin Shin Do Bodymind Acupressure, has been on faculty at the Connecticut Center for Massage Therapy for 16 years, and was a four-year faculty member at the Kripalu Yoga Institute. She is licensed in the state of Connecticut, where she maintains a private practice, and is currently a fourth-year student of Naturopathic Medicine at the University of Bridgeport. Her real love is using acupressure to help abused, neglected, or injured horses. You can find classes with Synthia and other qualified professionals at www.bodymindeast.com and www.jinshindo.org.

Bobbi Dempsey is a freelance writer for many major publications including *The New York Times, Muscle & Fitness, Family Circle, Parents, Men's Fitness,* and many others. She is also the author of numerous nonfiction books on topics ranging from diabetes to homemade ice cream. Her Web site is www.magazine-writer.com.

Dedication

Synthia would like to dedicate this book to her mother, Susan Ramsby, who "taught us the truly important things in life and who has facilitated and supported every part of my path."

Authors' Acknowledgments

From Synthia: First and foremost, a big thank you to Colin, Erin, and Adriel, who support all my various projects. Deep gratitude to the teachers who put me on the acupressure path — Iona Marsaa Teeguarden, Debra Valentine Smith, and Jasmine Wolf. Also, huge thanks to Steven Spignesi and Mike Lewis for opening the door; to our editor Kristin DeMint for her unparalleled patience; and to Bobbi Dempsey for welcoming me into the project and teaching me the ropes.

From Bobbi: I would like to thank, first and foremost, my co-author Synthia Andrews for her dedication and tireless efforts in making this book the best it can be. Also, to Marilyn Allen for bringing everyone together, and to Kristin DeMint for all her valuable input and guidance. And, as always, to John, Nick, and Brandon for serving as my constant motivation.

Publisher's Acknowledgments

We're proud of this book; please send us your comments through our Dummies online registration form located at www.dummies.com/register/.

Some of the people who helped bring this book to market include the following:

Acquisitions, Editorial, and Media Development

Project Editor: Kristin DeMint

Acquisitions Editor: Michael Lewis

Copy Editor: Sarah Faulkner

Technical Editors:
Mitchell Harris, L.Ac, MSTOM, Dipl. OM; and Erica Joy Harris, L.Ac, MSTOM, Dipl. OM; www.indyacu.com

Medical Illustrator: Kathryn Born, M.A.

Senior Editorial Manager: Jennifer Ehrlich

Editorial Assistants: Leeann Harney, David Lutton, Erin Calligan Mooney, Joe Niesen

Cartoons: Rich Tennant
(www.the5thwave.com)

Composition Services

Project Coordinator: Erin Smith

Layout and Graphics: Carl Byers, Joyce Haughey, Stephanie D. Jumper, Alicia B. South

Anniversary Logo Design: Richard Pacifico

Proofreaders: Aptara, Susan Moritz, Christy Pingleton

Indexer: Aptara

Special Help
Christina Guthrie, Kathy Simpson, Carmen Krikorian

Publishing and Editorial for Consumer Dummies

Diane Graves Steele, Vice President and Publisher, Consumer Dummies

Joyce Pepple, Acquisitions Director, Consumer Dummies

Kristin A. Cocks, Product Development Director, Consumer Dummies

Michael Spring, Vice President and Publisher, Travel

Kelly Regan, Editorial Director, Travel

Publishing for Technology Dummies

Andy Cummings, Vice President and Publisher, Dummies Technology/General User

Composition Services

Gerry Fahey, Vice President of Production Services

Debbie Stailey, Director of Composition Services

Contents at a Glance

Table of Contents

Introduction

*F*ace it: Life is stressful. Just going through your normal daily routine can often leave you frazzled and out of balance. And, if you're like most people, you also have to cope with your share of aches and pains, ranging from those mild-yet-irritating annoyances to the big-time, all-consuming pains.

Wouldn't it be great if you could wave a magic wand to restore balance and harmony to your life and to help alleviate some of those aches and pains?

Well, in a way, you can. Only instead of a magic wand, you use your own two hands (or someone else's). That's all it takes to unleash the healing power you have inside you — power that you can put to good use through the techniques of acupressure and reflexology.

About This Book

Because acupressure and reflexology are rooted in ancient oriental healing arts, they can seem mysterious and intimidating to understand. That's where this book comes in. We tell you everything you need to know about these bodywork techniques, from start to finish. We begin by explaining exactly what acupressure and reflexology are, and how they came to be. After a short history lesson (very brief, we promise), we get into the real "meat" of the book — showing you exactly how these techniques can improve your quality of life and alleviate some of your pain.

Conventions Used in This Book

To help you navigate easily through this book, we set up a few conventions that we use consistently throughout the book:

- Anytime we want to highlight new words or terms that we define in the text, we *italicize* them.
- **Boldfaced** text is used to indicate the action part of numbered steps and the keywords of a bulleted list.
- We use monofont for Web sites and e-mail addresses.

✔ In the illustrations and healing routines, we use abbreviations for the acupoints for simplicity's sake — we provide the full names of the points and their accompanying meridians (see Chapter 1 for a definition) in the accompanying tables.

✔ Every acupoint has many functions, and different routines use the same points for different reasons. We list only the functions that we're focusing on in a specific routine, so you see different functions for the same point in different routines.

✔ Because acupressure was developed in Japan from Chinese acupuncture theories and practices, the terms used to describe these two very similar practices are often different, which can cause some confusion. In this book, we use the Japanese terms. We do, however, provide the Chinese names as well in cases where the Chinese terms are more common.

✔ Some meridians have multiple names. In this book, we use the meridian names we like best.

✔ Most acupoints have many different names. We used the most common names in this book, but you may see many variations in other literature.

✔ The meridian illustrations throughout this book are renditions and aren't meant to be taken as exact maps. For precise detail, refer to acupuncture textbooks.

✔ The bladder meridian (see Chapter 3) has two different numbering systems. In this book, we use the system that numbers the inside line and then the outside line before heading down the leg. (Traditional Chinese Medicine, from which acupuncture stems, typically uses the alternate numbering system.)

When this book was printed, some Web addresses may have needed to break across two lines of text. If you come across these instances, rest assured that we haven't put in any extra characters (such as a hyphen) to indicate the break. So, when typing one of these Web addresses in a Web browser, just type in exactly what you see in this book, pretending as if the line break doesn't exist.

Foolish Assumptions

Although we normally don't like to make assumptions, we made an exception in this case in order to make this book most helpful to as many readers as possible. To that end, we assume that:

✔ You have little or no previous training in acupressure or reflexology.

✔ You have a positive attitude and will do your best to focus that positive energy on the healing process.

✔ You approach this process with an open mind, welcoming new ideas and techniques that may seem strange or foreign to you at first.

✔ You or someone you know has some aches, pains, or general uneasiness that you or they want to treat in a natural way.

✔ You want to discover how your body has the capability of healing itself (within reason — we'd *never* suggest that acupressure or reflexology can cure cancer or perform any other type of medical miracle).

What You're Not to Read

Granted, we like to think every single word on these pages is important. However, the information in the gray sidebars is interesting and informative, but it isn't required reading in order for to you to grasp the material in each chapter. We like to think of them as a bonus — a tasty little dessert to enjoy after you digest the main course.

How This Book Is Organized

Acupressure and Reflexology For Dummies is divided into five parts, each of which has its own special theme and focus. Here's an outline of the parts, and highlights of what you can find in each of them.

Part 1: Touching on the Basics of Acupressure and Reflexology

If you know little or nothing about these bodywork techniques, we recommend that you start by reading Part I. Here, we give you all the basics of these healing arts, including

✔ Definitions of important terms

✔ A quick overview of the history of ancient oriental healing arts

✔ Basic healing art principles such as qi, yin/yang, and energy forces

✔ Things you need to know to prepare to heal yourself or others

✔ Maps of the meridians and reflex zones, the foundations of these healing sessions, to serve as your guide throughout the rest of the book

✔ Full explanations of all the techniques used in both acupressure and reflexology, along with illustrations to show you how to perform them

This part also teaches some basic exercises that come in handy to get you warmed up, and gives you a preview of what the recipient and provider can both expect from a session. We also cover all the important issues you need to consider when enlisting professional help — from finding qualified candidates to evaluating their credentials. In addition, we give you a sneak peek of what to expect from your first session.

Part II: Promoting Emotional and Physical Wellness

An important concept when it comes to healing is the strong connection between emotional health and physical well-being. If your emotions are upset or out of balance, you will almost inevitably experience physical discomfort as a result. This is a major belief in the healing arts. Separating emotional and physical well-being is almost impossible. The two go hand-in-hand, and if you focus on one while neglecting the other, you won't reap the full benefits of your healing sessions.

To that end, in this part we focus on maintaining the best possible health, both physically and emotionally. We explain the correlation between energy and emotions, and we show you how negative and positive thinking can affect your physical well-being.

Of course, we know that realistically you can't totally avoid emotional stress, so we also show you how to do damage control and keep those unavoidable stressors from wreaking havoc on your body.

Part III: Where Does It Hurt? Treating Common Aches and Ailments

Most likely, you're dealing with at least one or two aches or pains at this very moment. Perhaps that's why you picked up this book, hoping it would help you attain some relief from your discomfort.

Relax, we're here to help. In this part, we target specific body parts and identify common ailments that often afflict those areas. More importantly, we provide — in clear, easy-to-understand steps — routines you can do to address these particular ailments.

Here are a few of the problems we cover in this part: backaches, including sciatica and muscle strain; pain in the hips and legs; headaches and other problems in the facial region; problems in the arms, shoulders, and hands; digestive problems and other stomach concerns; and issues affecting the heart and chest.

Part IV: Addressing Specific Needs and Concerns

In this part, we get a bit more specific, addressing issues that may be of particular interest to certain groups of people.

First, we touch on the various pains and problems that tend to be age related. This applies to people on all ends of the chronological spectrum, from babies to seniors and everyone in between.

Then we discuss those myriad problems that plague our female readers. Ladies, we feel your pain — and we come to your rescue in Chapter 16. (To our male readers: We're not neglecting you. It's just that women have several major gender-specific needs, whereas the majority of problems that may plague men are covered throughout other areas of this book.)

We also cover routines for handling common conditions like colds and the flu, and we talk about boosting the immune system for preventive measures.

Part V: The Part of Tens

In every *For Dummies* book, you find the Part of Tens. The last two chapters in this book address facts and fallacies about acupressure and reflexology, and also illustrate just a few of the many ways that these healing arts can enrich your life.

And last but not least, we include an appendix full of various resources in case you hunger for a more advanced understanding of acupressure and reflexology, want to find a good practitioner, or simply want to talk it up with others who love the healing arts as much as you do.

Icons Used in This Book

Throughout this book, you find different small pictures in the margins. These pictures, called *icons,* alert you to little tidbits of information along the way.

Here's a list of icons you will encounter in this book:

As the name implies, this icon lets you know that we're sharing a little helpful piece of information that relates in some way to the material we cover in that section.

This icon points out little pieces of material that you should commit to memory.

You should pay special attention to the Warning icon, because it cautions you away from things you should avoid in order to stay safe and prevent any problems.

Where to Go from Here

Although we hope you find this book so intriguing that you devour it from cover to cover, the path you take to explore it is totally up to you. We designed this book to be a complete how-to guide for the beginning healer. If you have a specific need, you can dive right into a specific chapter. The chapters are complete and thorough enough to stand on their own so that you can zero in on particular topics (or parts of the body) that interest you most.

Otherwise, we recommend starting at the beginning and working your way through the book. Don't worry — you can jump past any topics that don't interest you at the moment and skip ahead to others that do. (You can always go back and catch up on what you missed later on.)

Part I
Touching on the Basics of Acupressure and Reflexology

The 5th Wave   By Rich Tennant

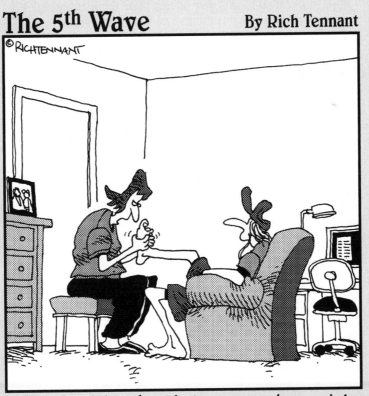

"What I'm doing should clear your sinuses, take away your headache, and charge your iPod."

In this part . . .

Part I gives you all the important essentials you need to know about acupressure and reflexology. Think of this as your Healing 101 introductory course.

We explain exactly what acupressure and reflexology are, and what they mean to anyone who needs emotional and/or physical healing. We fill you in on the history of the healing arts and the meaning of *qi*. We tell you what you need to heal yourself and others — your own two hands and confidence in yourself — and give you a little pep talk to strengthen your faith in your innate ability to heal.

Finally, we review the anatomical concepts that you need to know in order to properly perform the techniques in this book. You become familiar with the meridians, acupoints, reflex zones, different types of tissue, and other body parts that play an important part in the healing process. Unless you already have some massage training, we strongly suggest that you read this part so that you know all the basics.

Chapter 1

Acupressure and Reflexology Essentials

In This Chapter

▶ Defining acupressure and reflexology

▶ Tracing the roots of the healing arts

▶ Getting the keys to understanding qi

▶ Finding out how bodywork can help you

*I*f you're like most people, you know little (if anything) about acupressure and reflexology. You may incorrectly believe that acupressure involves needles. It doesn't — but don't worry, we address that and other misconceptions in the next few chapters. And when thinking about reflexology, you may guess from the name that it involves your reflexes in some way, but that may pretty much be the extent of your insight on the topic.

Or perhaps you *do* have some knowledge of the healing arts. You may know, for example, that a basic tenet of these approaches is the idea that pain can often be traced back to its root, which is often some distance away from the place where the pain is felt. However, you may not know exactly what that is, or how to trace the source of your pain.

Regardless of your knowledge level, or your reason for wanting to discover more, you can definitely benefit from reading about these important approaches to healing. Bodywork is beneficial to almost everyone, and it's often helpful if you know the background behind the techniques.

In this chapter, you explore the roots of reflexology and acupressure. You find out about the fundamental principles involved, including the concept of qi. Finally, and perhaps most importantly, you discover how these approaches to healing can help *you*. No matter what your physical ailment or health concern, you'll probably be pleasantly surprised at the difference even a minimal amount of bodywork can make.

Acupressure and Reflexology Defined

Before you get too far into the healing routines and practices that we discuss in this book, you need to make sure that you understand exactly what acupressure and reflexology are. They're closely related, and in much of this book we refer to them jointly as a pair of complementary healing arts. But despite their similarities, they do have some differences.

Acupressure

Acupressure is an ancient healing art that entails using an object (generally the hands or arms) to stimulate specific key points on the body with the goal of relieving pain or discomfort. Pain and discomfort are considered to be signs of energy imbalance, which, if left in this state, will become illness and disease.

Acupressure approaches this energy imbalance in a concrete way through the identification of *acupoints*. Acupoints are located on *meridians,* or channels that run throughout the body and connect all parts of the body together. These acupoints are specific sites on the body that often treat pain or discomfort elsewhere. By addressing problems or imbalances at the acupoints, you can balance the flow of energy and thereby reduce or eliminate pain in the affected areas.

Many people confuse acupressure with *acupuncture.* The two are similar and closely related. Both rely on the same fundamental principles, and both use the same points and meridians. The most important difference: acupuncture uses pins — technically, they're hair-thin, sterile needles — and acupressure doesn't. This difference is crucial, because the needle aspect is something that makes many people squeamish or nervous about acupuncture. For those people, acupressure can be an equally effective — yet much less nerve-wracking — alternative.

Eunice Ingham: Reflexology's patron saint

Reflexology first began catching on in the United States in the early 1900s. This was due in large part to a woman named Eunice Ingham. Eunice was a massage therapist who worked in the 1920s for a man named Joe Shelby Riley. Dr. Riley was well known as the creator of the Zone Theory, which is often seen as the precursor to modern-day reflexology. Inspired by Dr. Riley, Eunice expanded on the ideas of zone therapy while focusing on only one zone, the feet. She published her first book on the topic, called *Stories the Feet Can Tell,* in 1938. Soon Eunice became an in-demand teacher and lecturer who was often asked to share her knowledge of healing therapies. Eventually, she was joined by her nephew, Dwight Byers, who went on to become the founder of the International Institute of Reflexology.

Reflexology

Reflexology is a system of healing based on balancing energy by stimulating areas in the feet and hands that relate to organs, glands, and parts of the body. Reflexology is similar to acupressure in basic principle, but the two have some differences as well. They both correct imbalances in the energy force by focusing on specific areas of the body where they pinpoint (and treat) that imbalance. Although acupressure involves meridians and acupoints, reflexology relies on pathways called *reflex zones,* which contain *reflex areas* located on the hands and feet. The reflex areas on the hands and feet are essentially holograms of the whole body; therefore, stimulating the hands and feet affects the whole body. By applying pressure to specific reflex points, you adjust the flow of energy and can create a positive response (reduced pain) in a corresponding location elsewhere on the body.

Digging Deeper into Origins and Philosophy

Many healing arts, including acupressure and reflexology, are based on the beliefs of Chinese energy medicine — which people first practiced more than 5,000 years ago. The ancient Chinese believed that spiritual imbalances caused many illnesses and physical ailments. In order to effectively address the pain, the Chinese believed, you needed to resolve your spiritual imbalance and get your energies and life force in a balanced state. In other words, the Chinese felt that you couldn't properly treat physical pain unless you also addressed your spiritual issues and any imbalances in your energy force. In this section, we explain a bit more about where this belief started as well as a bit about how acupressure and reflexology support that philosophy.

The origins of acupressure and reflexology

Acupressure and reflexology are no New Age "flash in the pan" trends. In fact, they've actually been around for thousands of years. Their roots are believed to trace back to the ancient people of Asia, who realized the many benefits of strategic touch as part of a healing therapy routine. (In the case of reflexology, some evidence indicates that ancient Egyptians also practiced this type of healing therapy. Treating the body through the feet and hands has also been found in many indigenous healing systems. For example, Native Americans and Australian aborigines are both believed to have healing practices based on foot manipulation.)

Huang Di Nei Jing

One of the most well-known works related to ancient Chinese medicine is the *Huang Di Nei Jing,* which translates to *The Medical Classic of the Yellow Emperor.* This book, believed to date back to around 200 B.C., details the philosophy and techniques of acupuncture and other forms of medical treatment. In addition, it also covers other important topics such as astronomy, weather, and military operations.

The ancient people of Asia discovered that pressing specific points on the body can reduce or eliminate pain — often in locations elsewhere on the body. Chinese doctors began focusing on pressure points as a way to treat pain, fight illnesses, and encourage healing after injuries. These sessions, like many others developed by the Chinese of the period, were often used to treat soldiers who had been injured in various military conflicts.

Stone probes, found in Chinese tombs and believed to date back thousands of years, are believed by experts to be the first tools used in acupuncture and acupressure. These stones were called *Bian stones* and were used as tools to apply pressure to acupoints.

Originally, in Asia, many schools of Chinese medicine passed down in family lines. Most of these schools were similar to each other, but they also had lots of little differences — such as the exact function, name, or location of a point, how you use point combinations, and the use of extra points and extra channels of qi. After the Maoist revolution, General Mao combined all the teachings into one, eliminating all the differences, and he called it *Traditional Chinese Medicine,* or TCM. However, current practices still use acupuncture and acupressure techniques that fall outside of TCM and don't necessarily use organ meridians or standard acupoints. Some examples are auricular (ear) acupuncture, which many practitioners use today to treat addictions, and Korean hand acupuncture, which is similar to reflexology. The point? These examples show the vast array of healing techniques available to practitioners who use acupressure and reflexology therapies.

How and why they work

The foundation of Chinese energy medicine is the belief that a balanced and positive energy force is imperative for good health and emotional well-being. If you move or manipulate this energy to create a more balanced harmonious state, they believed you could effectively treat pain and illness.

As many people now acknowledge, the ancient Chinese healers were on to something. Today, people know that the body is like a big puzzle, with each part interconnected to other parts in many different (and sometimes mysterious) ways. In other words, you may say, "No man's body part is an island." A problem that originates with one part of the body inevitably begins to have repercussions on other parts of the body and mind.

Determining Preference: It's Up to You

We use acupressure and reflexology together in this book because the effects of one reinforce the effects of the other (see Chapter 3 for more detail). We can't give you a magic formula that tells you when using acupressure would be more beneficial than using reflexology. Many times it's a matter of preference — maybe you want to have your whole body touched and like the full-body approach of acupressure. Or maybe you have ticklish feet. Everyone is a little different, and some people respond better to one type of session than the other. Most people, however, enjoy both, and adding both to a session is the ideal because you're impacting more than one pathway and stimulating more than one type of physiological effect.

You may notice more acceptance of acupressure than reflexology in the mainstream. The reason? Acupressure has been studied more by Western medicine. Although Russians have studied reflexology, it has largely been ignored by medical researchers in the West. This fact is surprising because according to the Pacific Institute of Reflexology, the founder of modern day reflexology, Dr. William Fitzgerald, was a specialist in Boston City Hospital; the Central London Ear, Nose and Throat Hospital in England; and the St. Francis Hospital in Hartford. Unfortunately, until scientific research validates this approach, reflexology won't reach the same level of acceptance as acupressure.

Fundamental Principles of Acupressure and Reflexology

Learning basic acupressure and reflexology is much easier when you understand the fundamental principles. Pressure point therapies don't work with your body as if it's a machine; they work with your body as an energy system. The energy involved is called *qi* (pronounced *kee*) or *chi* (pronounced *chee*). Health and healing is dependent on the smooth and abundant flow of qi throughout the body. Life events can challenge your energy system, disrupting the flow of qi and causing imbalance.

Pressure point therapies seek to regain balance. Pressure is applied to specific points to regulate the flow of qi. As qi becomes more balanced, healing processes are stimulated. In this section, we focus on how this works and what forces are involved.

Your body as an energy system: An Eastern approach to healing

You probably know that models of healing in the West are significantly different from those in the East. In the West, health practitioners see the body as a machine. When the machine has a breakdown, medicine fixes the symptoms and considers that health has been restored. The progression is linear, and goes something like this:

1. **You get sick.**

2. **You have symptoms.**

3. **You stop the symptoms.**

4. **You feel better.**

Treatment is goal oriented, and the goal is to eliminate symptoms. Here's an example: You go to the doctor with heartburn. Using Western medicine, she gives you an antacid or a drug to block the production of acid. With either treatment your symptoms go away, and her job is done, even though the cause of the problem may not be addressed.

In the East, health practitioners see the body as an energy system. The progression of illness goes something like this:

1. **Your energy flow is disrupted.**

2. **You develop symptoms that show you where the energy imbalance is located.**

3. **Treatment involves shifting the cause of the imbalance.**

Treatment focuses on patterns and cycles of disease. Rather than being goal oriented, Eastern medicine tries to understand what the symptoms mean. Here's an example in this model: You go to the doctor with heartburn, and he assesses the balance and flow of your qi. He determines that the symptoms reveal too much qi in your stomach. He uses pressure point therapies to stimulate the rebalancing of qi and to explore the underlying patterns that created the imbalance. Are you working too much? Do you consistently burn the candle at both ends? Is this overwork an attempt to feel more useful, more worthy of recognition? After you understand your pattern, pressure point therapy can more effectively stimulate qi. Why? Because your mind and emotions are no longer working against you. Now that the pattern is shifted and your qi is balanced, you no longer need the symptoms of heartburn to tell you that you're out of balance.

Results-based payments for Chinese doctors

In ancient China, every village had a doctor. The doctor's job was to prevent illness and keep everyone in the village healthy. Each month, the doctor was paid for his services, but only if everyone stayed healthy. If anyone got sick, they considered the illness a failure on the doctor's part, and the doctor didn't get paid — now that's preventive medicine! Today it's up to you to practice preventive medicine and stay healthy — the doctor gets paid only when people get sick. And one of the most effective ways that you can keep yourself healthy (in addition to maintaining healthy nutrition and regular exercise, of course) is to use acupressure and/or reflexology. The tools and techniques in this book can go a long way toward keeping your qi balanced, your body and mind healthy, and your doctor bills low! Co-author Synthia has been practicing them for years, so trust her on this one.

In the Western model, the doctor does the healing. Your body heals, but the doctor does it! In the Eastern view, you already have everything you need to heal yourself. All body processes are geared toward self-healing. Pressure point therapies help shift patterns to remove obstacles to balance. Everything is based on timing. You can't force someone else's energy to change, and you don't know the best timing for change to happen. When giving yourself or someone else a healing session, you're facilitating change. Whether or not that change happens is up to the wisdom of the body. Never try to force results. Daylight can't come until night is over.

The importance of qi

Unfortunately, we can't give you an exact definition of qi. Trying to define it is like trying to define consciousness or infinity. They aren't easily and intuitively grasped, but they're the foundations of higher principles. Essentially, *qi* is life force, but Chinese texts describe it not only as a force, or energy, but also as a substance. It's a substance that acts through matter, binding molecules together, organizing them into form, and holding form together. At the same time, it's a force that enlivens and activates the form it organizes.

Qi can be described as vital force that sustains all life. Have you heard the expression "dead weight"? That's a body without qi flow. Consider two bodies with all their structures working properly: one is alive and one is dead. The presence or absence of vital life force is the only difference between the two.

Every culture has a concept and name for life force. In China it's chi; in Japan it's qi or ki; in India it's prana; Polynesians call it mana; in Hebrew it's rauch; Islamic cultures call it barraka; and Native American and Australian tribes all have different names as well. In modern times, people have referred to it as biomagnetism, plasma, orgone, L-fields, and factor X.

The duality of light

The description of qi as both energy and matter is very similar to the duality of light. Isaac Newton described light as a particle and designed experiments that proved it. His contemporary Christian Huygens described light as a wave and designed experiments that proved this, too. It took almost two centuries before people began to accept that light is both a particle (matter) and a wave (energy), expressing itself differently under different conditions. Understanding the duality of light gave rise to quantum physics. Were the ancient Chinese aware of this duality centuries earlier?

Where does qi come from?

Qi is everywhere. It's present within, between, and around everything that exists. You can think of it as an ocean of qi that you're swimming within (and don't forget, humans are 65 percent water — or in this case, qi!). You may hear people call it universal life force or universal qi. Universal qi changes form when it embodies matter and becomes an individualized life force. You may not know it, but you were born with your own personalized qi that's yours for life. You may be asking yourself right now whether you were born with enough qi to last you your entire life. The truth is that you spend qi every day. Every activity you perform (including thinking!) uses qi. To live a long and healthy life, you need an abundance of qi, so supplementing your original qi is important.

Keeping your qi plentiful

You restock your qi in three different ways. The first way is to obtain qi from the world around you through the air you breathe, through the food you eat, and through natural elements like sunlight. The quality of qi you have to live your life with depends on the quality of what you eat and the environment you're in. Take a minute to consider the quality of qi that's becoming you. Is it reflected in the quality of your health, thoughts, and emotions?

Another way you replenish your qi is to generate it internally. Many systems have been developed to generate internal qi. Yoga, T'ai Chi, and Qi Kung are three moving methods of generating internal energy. Pranic breathing and mediation practices are two of the more sedentary approaches. Your ability to generate internal qi is affected by your thoughts and emotions. Do the thoughts you think give you more energy, or do they drain your energy? You may want to try one of these practices to build your internal energy reserves. Two good books to get you started are *T'ai Chi For Dummies,* by Therese Iknoian, and *Yoga For Dummies,* by Georg Feuerstein and Larry Payne (both published by Wiley).

A third way to supplement qi is through connection to universal qi. All the methods that teach you how to generate internal energy ultimately help you to connect with universal qi. As you become more and more attuned to universal qi, you can begin to fill directly from the source, keeping your own supply vibrant and abundant.

What does qi do?

Talking about what qi does is easier than talking about what qi is. All your cells need to be nourished and sustained with life force. Without life force, your cells would be, well, lifeless! Life force organizes the development of your body, animates you, and motivates you. Without qi, your body degenerates and decomposes; with a deficiency of qi, your life may lack meaning and direction, and your body may lack vibrant health. Qi provides your *body-mind* (a common term illustrating that the body and mind are so interconnected that they really should be treated as one) with information, directing your cells and psyche in fulfilling your own unique design. Not to be overlooked, qi is also a connecting force, connecting your organs, teeth, and tissue to each other; your mind to your body; and your spirit to your path. As it connects you internally, it connects you externally, allowing you to feel attached to the world you live in.

Accepting that qi codes and transmits information is often hard. However, information is always transmitted on energy carrier waves. For example, you access information encoded onto radio waves and microwaves every time you turn on your radio or use your cellphone.

The bottom line? Qi keeps you healthy. When qi is flowing unrestricted through your body, it harmonizes all organs and optimizes body functioning. Have you ever experienced the hum of feeling on top of the world; feeling vibrant, alive, and where you're supposed to be in the universe? This is the feeling of unrestricted, free-flowing, and balanced qi! Using pressure point therapies can help you find this internal balance.

Meridians, acupoints, and reflex points as conductors of qi

Qi is organized in the body in channels called *meridians.* These channels distribute qi to every organ, tissue, and cell in your body. They start as large channels and branch into smaller and smaller channels. You can think of it like arteries becoming arterioles and then capillaries, delivering blood to the cells. Another useful comparison is to think of them like streams or irrigation channels. All supply vital nutrients that are needed for health. Meridians have a higher conductivity than surrounding tissue.

Acupoints are points on the meridians that are closest to the surface of the skin (although some are deeper, depending on where they're located on the body). They have an even higher conductivity to energy flow than the rest of the meridian; this energy flow can be measured with micro-electrical voltage meters attached to the skin. Consequently, acupoints are like little whirlpools in a stream. Pressing these whirlpool points helps to regulate the flow of qi.

Reflexology also works with life energy, but it doesn't focus on the meridians as transporters of qi. Pressing the *reflex points* on the feet and hands influences qi reflexively. You push a point on the feet that relates to an organ, and, through a reflexive action, qi flow to the organ is increased or decreased as needed. Although reflexology doesn't focus on meridians, many meridians start or end in the feet, which may be another reason why reflexology can be so effective.

How qi imbalance affects health

So how do acupressure or reflex points get empty or full? Imbalance can happen in several ways. Energy flow is impacted by injury, overuse, poor nutrition, emotional trauma, pain, being in bad environments, stress, pollution, and toxic overload, to name a few. When imbalance happens, energy accumulates in some areas and is depleted in other areas. Areas of accumulation can become stagnant, like blood pooling in the extremities. Stagnant qi loses its energetic quality and the ability to promote health. Areas of depletion become isolated, losing access to healthy qi flow and losing connection to the rest of the body.

Imbalance in the qi flow impacts your health in many ways. It can open the door to the development of disease, it can give you muscle tension and pain, or it can cause you to feel depression or anxiety. If you've had an imbalance for a long time, you may experience loss of function or a lowered immune system. Maybe you have a small or relatively new imbalance; in that case, you probably feel just a little off or under the weather. Whether you have a big imbalance or a little imbalance, you can support your health by regulating qi flow with pressure point therapies.

Emotions, the mind, and qi

Where you put your attention influences where your qi flows. Are you thinking all the time about how bad you feel or how tired you are? Guess what? You're instructing your qi to maintain the status quo! And you could be causing more qi to become obstructed or depleted. Instead, try generating some internal qi, and then practice sending it to the areas in your body that need it. How do you do that? By focusing your attention on areas that need help and imagining life force flowing to those areas. If you have life force (and if you're reading this, you should!), it will follow your attention and support your body in achieving better health.

The heart is considered the seat of Shen, or your spirit. When you're in a healthy state, your mind follows the mandates of your spirit, the heart of who you are. Your emotions are your body's way of translating the desires of the heart. Every emotion is linked to a specific organ and has a defined function. Some emotions calm the qi, and some emotions disrupt the qi. All emotions are normal responses to life events and have value. However, if you get stuck in a specific emotional pattern, your qi flow can be disrupted.

Do you find that you always react the same way? Maybe you feel irritable a lot, or you say no to every question, or maybe you say yes to everything even when you don't want to. Maybe everything scares you so that you never want to go places and do things. These situations are examples of being stuck in an old emotional pattern that disturbs your flow of qi. You can read more about emotions — and find some exercises to balance your emotional qi — in Chapters 7 and 8. Every thought you think and every emotion you feel directs your energy.

Yin and yang: Forces of health

The yin/yang symbol is the fundamental expression of Eastern medicine and philosophy. You've probably already seen this symbol in many different places (if you haven't, check out Figure 1-1). It's a circle divided in two; one side is a swirl of black (yin) and the other side is a swirl of white (yang). The black swirl contains a white dot, and the white swirl contains a black dot, indicating that within each is the seed of the other. But what does this symbol mean, and what does it have to do with pressure point therapy?

Figure 1-1:
The yin/yang symbol of balance and harmony.

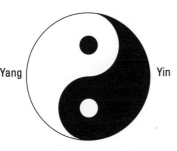

Yang   Yin

Yin and yang are the two opposing forces of the universe. Although they're opposites, they're not unrelated; they're different halves of the same whole or different sides of the same coin. You can't have one without the other. You can't have a mountain without a valley, or day without night, and you can't have yin without yang. All things are composed and contain both yin and yang — matter, qi, and even emotions. When something contains more yin than yang, it's considered to be yin, and vice-versa — but never forget that both aspects are still present in all things.

The qualities of yin are considered to be feminine, and the qualities of yang are considered to be masculine (see the nearby sidebar "Qualities of yin and yang" for more info). Yin and yang exist only in relation to each other; nothing is yin or yang all by itself — it can be yin or yang only in relation to something else. For example: If yang is hot and yin is cold, then what's warm — yin or yang? If you're comparing warm to cold, warm is yang. If you're comparing warm to hot, warm is yin. Warm by itself is neither or both.

Health is the dynamic balance between yin and yang forces in the body. Sometimes a person needs more yang energy. Remember the time you had to stay up all night painting a new room? Without activating yang energy, you wouldn't have been able to do it. Sometimes a person needs more yin energy. Remember how long it took to recover from staying up all night? Without nurturing yin energy, you wouldn't have been able to recover! The ability to respond to what's needed in a situation is a keynote of good health.

When you're using pressure point therapy, you determine your healing routine based on whether the points are yin or yang (empty or full). You can determine that a point is yin or yang only in comparison with another point, and we show you how in Chapter 4.

The Tao of change

Tao loosely translates as *the way* or *the path*. However, it doesn't mean one way or one path, but the way or the path of the individual. Other translations are *the origin of all things, the way of nature,* and *the ultimate reality.* In the yin/yang symbol, the Tao is represented by the circle, symbolizing all that is. The Tao divides itself into two opposite expressions, yin and yang; the dynamic tension between yin and yang creates qi, the energy and substance of all that exists within the Tao.

Take a good look back at Figure 1-1. You may notice that as one swirl gets bigger, the other gets smaller. In fact, when the yin side gets as big as it can, it flips and becomes the yang side, which starts small and gets bigger and bigger until it too flips and becomes the yin side. Yin and yang aren't static. They're constantly moving, turning one into the other; night turns into day, and winter turns into spring. Change is a constant in the universe. Staying the same isn't possible. Change, however, isn't random — it happens when the timing is right; morning only comes when night is finished. This notion is important in the practice of acupressure.

Qualities of yin and yang

Yin and yang are each associated with specific qualities. For example:

✔ **Qualities of yin:** Cold, dark, night, earth, incubation, moon, rest, contraction, soft, deficient, empty, matter, nurturing, calm

✔ **Qualities of yang:** Hot, light, day, heaven, creation, sun, activity, expansion, hard, excessive, full, energy, defensive, passionate

---

Health, like the Tao, is always changing. It's a dynamic equilibrium between the forces of yin and yang. If health was a static state, you wouldn't be able to respond to changing situations and environmental demands.

So, all these fundamentals are interesting, but do you need to know them to perform pressure point therapies? Well, the answer is yes and no. You can certainly give pressure point sessions knowing nothing about the dynamic forces you're working with, and you can even be effective. On the other hand, understanding these principles will assist you in giving the most effective sessions possible, assessing the needs of the person you're working with, and minimizing uncomfortable side effects.

Personalizing the Benefits and Cautions

Even if you have a good understanding of the basic principles of acupressure and reflexology (if you don't, just check out the earlier parts of this chapter), you still may be thinking, "That's all very interesting — but how can these techniques help *me* personally?"

That answer varies depending on your specific situation and any health concerns you have. But the general answer is that bodywork can help you in many ways by improving your overall health and well-being and alleviating pain while treating any illnesses or nagging injuries you may have. This, in turn, will surely improve your emotional health and spiritual harmony.

What acupressure and reflexology can do for you

The following list looks at a few specific ways in which acupressure and reflexology may be able to help you:

✔ **Immune support:** Bodywork therapies can have a major positive impact on your immune system. The ancient Chinese believed that too much (or too little) energy in a certain meridian or zone could cause undue stress, which would weaken the immune system.

Although specific acupoints are often cited as being specific "immune booster" targets, addressing any energy imbalances you may have will certainly have a positive impact on the state of your immune system.

For maximum benefit to your immune system, use healing arts in conjunction with related techniques, such as meditation and deep breathing. In addition, avoid stress whenever possible.

Also, using bodywork techniques to treat any specific condition you may have — say, a cold or sinus infection — will alleviate the toll on your immune system.

✔ **Circulatory stimulation:** One of the basic goals of bodywork techniques is to stimulate the proper circulation of energy. But here's a little secret: blood flow follows energy. So, in essence, by opening pathways for energy, you simultaneously stimulate blood to flow better.

Acupressure and reflexology are excellent ways to stimulate your circulatory system, which is essential to good health. Poor circulation can cause all sorts of undesirable problems, from cramps and swelling (especially in the legs and feet) to more serious conditions like blood clots and strokes.

In addition, poor circulation makes it tougher for your body to heal areas that have suffered a wound or other injury.

✔ **Relieving aches, pains, and muscle strains:** Bodywork is perhaps most well-known (and most commonly employed) as an effective way to treat aches and pains. Although any type of massage or muscle stimulation (if done properly) can help alleviate aches and pains, the techniques used in acupressure and reflexology can allow you to pinpoint the root of the pain, thus treating it much more quickly and efficiently.

Plus, by using these techniques correctly, you can often treat pain in several different parts of the body at once (or in rapid succession), thus providing a healing option that can save you considerable time and effort.

✔ **Rehabilitation and support for injury recovery:** Bodywork is also commonly used to help the body heal more quickly following an injury. By encouraging the optimal flow of energy to the affected area (and stimulating its corresponding acupoints), you can often speed up the healing and recovery process. In addition, eliminating or reducing pain in that area makes it much easier to perform physical therapy exercises or other routines involved in the rehabilitation process.

✔ **Optimal wellness and performance:** It's common knowledge that if you feel better, you perform better. Performing at your best (in sports, work, or anything else) is tough if you're plagued by pain or struggling with injuries.

Improving your energy flow not only helps the specific areas involved, but also boosts your overall well-being and puts you in a more positive frame of mind. This combination allows you to perform at your peak level, while also sustaining proper energy flow necessary for endurance.

✔ **Stress reduction:** One of the most important benefits of acupressure and reflexology is stress reduction. Restoring balance to the system reduces muscle tension and promotes relaxation. When you begin to change the patterns of imbalance, stress automatically reduces in your life.

✔ **Emotional growth and transformation:** During a pressure point session, you may experience deep relaxation. This type of relaxation allows you to access deeper places within. Here you may find some of the patterns that keep you from being fully satisfied in life. You may find that you're able to see things with a new perspective and that issues that have always bothered you don't anymore.

✔ **Making you aware that your body is your temple:** Universal qi is a pretty special substance. You store it in your body, so increasing internal qi sort of makes your body a temple. When this increase of internal qi happens, you may find that you develop a new appreciation for your body, for being alive, and for the special and unique place you have on this planet.

What injuries and ailments you need to avoid

Professionals are trained to work with different pathologies, but because you're just starting, stay away from pressure point therapy on the following conditions:

✔ Varicose veins, especially deep or painful conditions

✔ Inflammation, a sign of injury — signs are redness, swelling, heat, and dysfunction

✔ Severe swelling (edema)

✔ Fractures, sprains, strains, or surgery

✔ Contagious diseases

✔ Infections

✔ Contusions, bruises, or bleeding

✔ Herniated disk in the spine

✔ Severe neck trauma

✔ Deep emotional issues or trauma

Supplementing and Complementing Acupressure and Reflexology

As you've probably realized by now, acupressure and reflexology can benefit your health and well-being in many ways. And even if your healing plan consists of these techniques alone, you're bound to see a noticeable improvement in the way you feel.

However, your results will be many times greater if you incorporate these techniques into a comprehensive overall treatment and lifestyle plan. For maximum benefit, you should supplement bodywork with other positive strategies, such as meditation, yoga, stretching, deep breathing, and related exercises. In addition, taking steps to reduce or eliminate stress will make a big difference in your health, both physically and mentally. Naturally, you should also practice other healthy-living habits — in other words, avoid smoking, maintain a healthy diet, exercise regularly, and get sufficient sleep.

All these healthy-living habits play an important role in how you feel and how your body performs. By bringing all these pieces together into one big treatment plan puzzle, you'll be amazed at the positive differences you see in your life.

Chapter 2

Healing Yourself or a Loved One

Chances are good that you're eager to rush right into a healing session, especially if you or a loved one is in pain right now. Your enthusiasm is understandable, but you must be patient. Before you just dive right in and practice these healing techniques, you need to spend a little time educating yourself about the basics of the process.

Consider all the important aspects of the healing process: why pain happens, what you can (and can't) realistically do about it, and the risks you need to keep in mind. Be prepared for the different sensations you may experience during a healing session. This preparation helps you avoid any unexpected (and possibly unwelcome) surprises.

The information in this chapter tells you how to become fully prepared before the session so that you can achieve the best results and maximum benefit.

Giving Yourself — or Others — a Healing Hand: The Basics

Anyone, at any time, can benefit from the techniques involved in bodywork. These healing strategies — whether self-administered or given to another — can relax and rejuvenate the body, and they're almost guaranteed to make you feel better, even if you're not in pain. However, people with pain or discomfort benefit the most from healing therapies. If you have aches, pains, sore muscles, or virtually any other source of physical discomfort, you're in need of a healing session. A weekend warrior still recovering from Saturday's football game? A healing session may be exactly what he needs. A busy mom whose back and legs ache from chasing after kids all day? She, too, should treat herself to a session, pronto.

Whether you plan to treat yourself or others, you just need to know the fundamentals of the healing arts. By simply brushing up on the basics of acupressure and reflexology, you can accomplish amazing results. Before you attempt to exert those powers on others, however, take care of the items on this list:

✔ Do some basic research (which you're doing right now by reading this book). This research ensures that you know the essentials of conducting a healing session.

✔ Make sure that the receiver is ready for the healing plan and able to experience a session safely. In the case of illness or injury, this step may involve consulting with a doctor before embarking on any healing plan.

The following sections explain what you need to know before deciding to treat yourself or someone else.

Benefits and drawbacks

You can find many benefits of participating in acupressure and reflexology. First and foremost, you probably feel better (possibly a lot better) after just the first session. Many people are pleasantly surprised at the noticeable improvement after their session.

Another benefit, if you perform a healing plan on yourself, is that you become much more in tune with your own body and the effect that healing sessions can have on it. This benefit gives you a boost of confidence in your power over pain and your ability to heal yourself or others. You may be amazed at the new revelations you discover about the connection between pain and its source(s). You may begin to see your body in an entirely new and fascinating way.

Healing sessions have few (if any) drawbacks if they're conducted properly. Obviously, you should use care and exert only enough pressure to perform the techniques without causing discomfort. Make sure that you're not using these techniques as a substitute for medical care and treatment. Serious illnesses and injuries need to be addressed by a doctor. Healing therapy should be applied in conjunction with a medical treatment plan, not in place of it.

When and where to get or provide a healing session

One of the best things about acupressure and reflexology is that you can use them virtually anywhere at anytime. You don't need elaborate, time-consuming preparations or a lot of expensive, bulky equipment. If you're treating yourself, all you really need is a peaceful space and your own two hands (a few tools may help, too; see the next section for suggestions). If you're treating someone else, you still need only your hands and a quiet moment. Of course, the ideal is to have a clean, quiet, comfortable space with no interruptions, but you can certainly help ease a headache by pressing points even when sitting on a busy bus. So don't hold back; use acupressure and reflexology when you need them!

When to start? The sooner, the better — especially if you're suffering from any kind of pain or discomfort. For best results, plan your acupressure and reflexology sessions for a time when you can concentrate without distractions. The exact timing often depends on your personality and preferences. Just as some people are night owls who like to conduct important tasks in the wee hours of the night, most people find that they most enjoy sessions at certain times of the day. Many people like to schedule their sessions for right before bed so that they can take advantage of the relaxing nature of these healing sessions. Others find the sessions invigorating, and thus view them as the perfect way to start the day.

The frequency of sessions may also vary depending on your preferences. You may experience a bit of soreness or sensitivity following an intense session. If so, you may want to wait a day or two before your next session. On the other hand, some people treat themselves to numerous mini-sessions several times throughout the day, and this practice isn't unusual. The important thing is to let your body be your guide and do whatever feels best for you.

Reaching those difficult places

If you're treating yourself, you can easily reach all the reflexology points and many of the acupressure points; however, some of the acupressure points require a bit of twisting and stretching; and still others may not be reachable at all! You may wish that you needed acupressure only on the easy points, but most people want to reach the points on the back the most. That's when a few tools can come in handy. Here are a couple of suggestions:

✔ **Two tennis balls and a sock:** The easiest and perhaps best tool you can ever have is simply made up of two tennis balls and a sock. Put the tennis balls in the sock all the way to the toe, and then tie the end of the sock so that the balls are held tightly together. Voilà — an acupressure tool! Simply place this tool of advanced technology between your back and the floor when lying down, or lean against a wall with the sock between your back and the wall (this technique works well when you want less pressure than your full body weight). Experiment by moving, rolling, and pressing to create the pressure you want on the areas you most need.

✔ **Professional acupressure tools for the back:** The best type of tool we've found for back acupressure points is anything with a knob ending on a curved or S-shaped rod. You can position the curve around your body or over your shoulder to place the knob exactly where you need it. A little leverage is all you need for just the right amount of pressure to feel the *ahh* of relief.

Of course, feet are pretty easy to reach — you probably need tools only if your thumbs get sore (this applies to both acupressure and reflexology). In that case, you may want to try any of the hand-held acupressure tools with knobby ends. They allow you to apply pressure but still give your thumbs a break. General stimulation on your feet is also good, and you can buy lots of rollers and massage mats for pressure point stimulation of the feet.

You can easily find acupressure tools on the Internet — simply perform a search, using Massage Tools or Acupressure Tools as your keywords.

Pain as part of healing

The body has an interesting response to injury. Have you ever had a sprained ankle? As soon as the ankle swells with inflammation and pain starts, the muscles all around the injury tighten up. This tightening is called *muscle splinting,* and it's the body's effort to immobilize the injury to prevent more damage. Sometimes the body forgets to relax the muscles and unsplint the area after the injury starts to get better. Unfortunately, this tends to stop the healing process, leaving weakened tissue, trigger points, and energy blocks in the meridians.

Healing techniques can restart the healing process by shifting the energy block and bringing energy into the area. When energy flows, circulation follows. Before you know it, the muscles are relaxing and the old injury is waking up! Although it may feel bad, this is a great sign that healing processes are underway and pain-free function is around the corner.

Setting reachable goals and expectations

Although ancient healing arts like reflexology and acupressure can have an air of mystery about them, they aren't magic and can't perform miracles. Keep your expectations realistic; otherwise, you may find yourself disappointed and tempted to give up before you make any real progress. Although you're likely to feel some level of relief almost immediately, using acupressure and reflexology is often a gradual process, and it can take a while to reach a point where your pain is really "conquered." This scenario is especially true in the case of chronic pain. After all, chronic pain didn't show up overnight, and expecting it to go away that quickly is unrealistic.

Granted, some people do experience amazingly quick relief following these healing sessions. Counting on that, however, is setting your expectations too high. Hope for just a moderate improvement, and then you can be pleasantly surprised if the results exceed your expectations.

So, what are reasonable goals and expectations? Simply put, your main goal for yourself or your receiver should be to feel increasingly better (even if only a little bit) after each session.

More exact goals depend upon specific pains or concerns. For example, if the pain in your legs makes sleeping difficult for you, one of your primary goals may be to get an uninterrupted night of sleep. A short-term goal may be to wake up less often and get more restful sleep than you were. *Note:* You may also notice that you're sleeping better because of the relaxing properties of bodywork.

The presence of pain — when no underlying injury is being aggravated and the receiver is in a comfortable position — gives good information about the health and energy flow (or lack thereof) in an area. If everything is physically okay, the pain may be the effects of increased qi (see Chapter 1 for more on qi) into a blocked area. Pain during a session usually decreases as the blocked energy begins to move, and you can continue working as long as the pain isn't excessive.

If the person you're treating feels increased pain, has an emotional release, or feels uncomfortable in some way during the session, use this information to direct the session and be more effective. Ask whether she wants less pressure or whether she wants to stop the session, but don't assume that she wants to stop or that what's happening is bad. Stay calm and centered and let the energy do its job. By staying calm and centered, you can allow healing space where your receiver can explore the blocks in his or her energy flow and maybe even shift them permanently. (See the later section "Achieving presence" for more on staying calm and centered.)

Good pain is the pain of healing. Bad pain is the pain of injury. Telling the difference can be difficult. Usually, good pain has an element of relief to it, and even though you feel sore, it hurts in good way. Good pain usually likes pressure and touch, doesn't last long, and gets better each day. Bad pain feels like damage is occurring. It may be red, hot, and angry feeling. It doesn't want to be touched and may get worse before it gets better.

Preparing Yourself to Give a Healing Session

Before you begin a healing session on yourself or someone else, spend some time preparing for it. You want to focus on locating the source of pain and then coming up with a healing plan and goal. Develop your presence by taking a few minutes to ground and center. Also, because this activity is physical, trying some of the stretches in the section "Staying fit" can help you become physically prepared for your session. Finally, pressure point therapy requires contact between you and your receiver. Be sure your fingernails are short and be aware of cleanliness.

Being prepared for the session means preparing your space, too. Having ready everything you require for the session is the last preparation you need. Be sure to have pillows or supports, maps and charts, music, and the healing plan you intend to use easily available.

Achieving presence

Have you ever used phrases such as "She was so scattered," or "He was all over the place"? These phrases describe people who are distracted and unfocused. Maybe they have too much on their minds, or maybe they've just received bad news. Although most people feel this way at one time or another, can you imagine giving a session feeling this way? Your session would be ineffective, and chances are good that you could hurt someone.

When giving someone a session, you must be fully present, focused on the person, and paying attention to the flow of the session. The quality of your attention is called *presence,* and your presence is the most important tool you have. Presence is what you project — the vibe you carry that people respond to.

Developing presence requires you to be grounded and centered. This concept sounds pretty esoteric, but it's really simple. Where you put your attention is where your energy flows. If your attention is scattered, your energy is scattered. If you want to be grounded, put your attention into the earth and your energy will follow. When you're grounded, you can easily stay balanced and relaxed no matter what you're doing or what's happening around you.

Maybe you're having a hard time making a decision, and your mind is flitting from one idea to the next, leaving you feeling uncentered. The solution? Bring your attention inward to the center of your body, to the area just below your belly button. This area is called the *hara* (in Japanese) or *Dan Tien* (in Chinese) and is the center of gravity in your physical body (we stick with the former in this book). When you bring your attention to your hara, your energy follows and you become more centered. Sound simple? It is! Being centered and grounded keeps you on track, and when you're on track, you make good decisions and give an effective session. It keeps you from getting over-involved and drained.

The language used in the fields of acupuncture and acupressure, two very similar healing arts, can be a bit confusing because acupuncture was developed in China, but acupressure was developed in Japan. So, acupuncture and acupressure terms aren't always in the same language! You don't need to know this info for this book, but if you deepen your study of acupressure, you should be aware that these nuances in language do exist.

Using a grounding exercise

The best way to become more grounded is to use your breath and your mind to direct your attention. As you breathe in, imagine your breath bringing energy into your body through the top of your head. Breathe this energy in and through your body. As you breathe out, imagine sending this energy out of your feet, deep into the earth, sending roots into the ground. In just a few short minutes you can enjoy the benefits of being grounded, which include greater focus and balance.

Homing in on a centering exercise

You can use your breath and mind to become more centered. Start by putting your right hand over your *hara* (the center of gravity in your physical body; it's under your belly button) and your left hand over your heart. As you breathe in, imagine your skin collecting light and pulling it in through all areas of your body. Imagine breathing this light through the center of your body and into your hara. With every breath in, let your energy build in your hara, moving up into your heart as well; with every breath out, release tension. You soon feel the clear, calming effects of being centered.

The hara is located one palm width down from your belly button and halfway between the front and back of your body. It's the biomechanical center of your body and the place where you store your excess qi. You can find more exercises on accessing your hara in Chapter 3.

Breathing into your belly (Hara breathing)

Expand your belly as you breathe in deeply and slowly, pulling air all the way down into the bottom of your abdomen. As you exhale, contract your abdominal muscles to push all the air out. Continue this breathing pattern five or six times with full and deep inhalations and complete exhalations. This technique helps build your energy as you ground and center.

Staying fit

Physical fitness is an important part of overall well-being, both for your body and your soul. If you're in good physical health, you feel better in every way and tend to have a more positive outlook on life.

Whole-body fitness is also important because it specifically relates to performing bodywork. If you're not in good physical shape, these techniques can quickly become tiring and may cause you to experience soreness and muscle aches.

Taking care of hands, arms, and shoulders

When you perform bodywork, your upper body (mainly your hands, arms, and shoulders) does the bulk of the work. Therefore, you should try to make sure those areas of your body are in the best possible shape so that you can perform these techniques as well as possible.

Your hands are your most important tool in acupressure and reflexology. Using them correctly ensures a long career in the healing arts. Using them incorrectly not only shortens your use in bodywork, but also affects all the other activities you use your hands for. Here are some tips for using your hands wisely:

✔ **Never use more pressure than is needed to release the point.** At first, knowing how much pressure to use is hard to pin down. With practice, you can feel things more clearly. When you're working points, ask yourself, "Can I maintain this amount of pressure using less muscle strength?" When starting out, practitioners of acupressure and reflexology commonly use more muscles to perform an action than are actually required. This is called *co-contraction* and can set you up for future injury.

Muscles that perform opposing actions are arranged opposite each other across a joint. For example, the muscles to straighten your knee cross the front of your knee joint, and the muscles that bend the knee cross the back of your knee joint. The same is true for the elbow, wrist, fingers, and all joints. Usually when one set of muscles contracts, the opposite set of muscles relaxes to allow the joint to move; if both sets of muscles contract (co-contraction), the joint can't move without a lot of effort to overcome the opposition. When applying pressure, new practitioners often co-contract, using way more muscle than they need!

✔ **Whenever possible, use reinforced fingers.** Using *reinforced fingers* means using more than one finger to apply pressure. If you're using your index finger to press the point, put your middle finger of the same hand behind your index finger to support your index finger.

✔ **Switch it up.** You're taught to apply pressure using lots of different parts of your hand and body, such as the knuckles, heel of the hand, elbows, and even knees. Switch the part you're using often to avoid overusing any one area.

✔ **Stretch your hands and wrists before, after, and during your sessions.**

✔ **If you have pain in your wrist or fingers after a session, you can ice them to decrease inflammation.** However, consider this pain a signal that you're using too much pressure in your sessions, or you're using your thumbs incorrectly. It's good to follow ice with gentle stretching to bring circulation and qi back into the joints. It's worth noting, though, that traditional Chinese medicine avoids the use of ice because it can cause stagnant qi, so be sure to keep the qi flowing with movement.

A good way to ice your hands or any hurting part is to put ice cubes in a plastic baggie until it's about one-third full. Add water to the level of the cubes. Squeeze out any air and close the bag. Wrap the bag in a wet, warm, thin towel and apply it to your hurting area. The warm towel will get cold, and you will go through four stages of sensation. First you will feel cold, then burning, then aching, then numbness. Keep the ice on until you feel numb or no longer than 20 minutes. This reduces inflammation, decreases pain, and stops spasms in muscles.

✔ **Stop when you're tired.** Consider acupressure or reflexology a sport and know that it takes time to strengthen your muscles for a new task.

✔ **Take a cue from professional massage therapists and use some of the specially designed massage tools available from a variety of retail stores and online retailers.** Both www.massagewarehouse.com and www.gaiam.com are good Web sites for purchasing tools and supplies.

Stretching the hands and arms

Taking care of your hands and arms is an essential part of giving a good session of acupressure and reflexology. This section gives you four easy stretches to do before you start.

This first exercise stretches your tricep and posterior deltoid muscles, both important in providing power to your work:

1. **Raise one arm over your head.**

2. **Bend the elbow of the arm over your head so that your hand falls toward your shoulder blades.**

3. **With your other hand, grasp your elbow and gently pull backward until you have a good, but comfortable, stretch.**

4. **Hold for 20 seconds.**

5. **Repeat on the other side.**

This exercise stretches your upper back, shoulder, and posterior arm muscles, keeping you from getting all bound up when working:

1. **Cross one arm over your chest.**

2. **With the other hand, grasp the elbow of your crossed arm and gently pull that arm farther across your chest.**

3. **Hold for 20 seconds.**

4. **Repeat on the other side.**

This exercise is very important in keeping the wrist flexible, allowing qi to flow freely into your hands:

1. **Place your palms together in front of your chest in prayer position.**

2. **If you comfortably can, gently raise your elbows toward the ceiling while keeping your palms connected.**

   Stop if you feel any pain in your wrists.

3. **Hold for 20 seconds.**

The final exercise for your hands and arms is the reverse of the exercise above; stretching the opposing muscles and keeping qi flowing smoothly:

1. **Place the backs of your hands together with your fingers pointing down.**

2. **Gently lower your elbows as far as you can.**

3. **Hold for 20 seconds.**

Benefiting from whole body stretching

You may also benefit from doing stretches that help increase the flexibility of your entire body. Following are some examples of basic simple stretches you may want to try.

This exercise stretches your back muscles:

1. **Lie on your back.**

2. **Bring your knees to your chest.**

3. **Hold your calves with your hands.**

4. **Hold for a moment, release, and repeat.**

If you want to stretch your legs, try this exercise:

1. **Stand upright with your feet wide apart.**

2. **Shift your body weight to one side.**

   Keeping your hands on your hips can help maintain balance.

3. **Bend from the waist to one side as far as you can without causing discomfort.**

4. **Reverse sides to stretch the other leg.**

If you're looking for another leg stretch, give this one a try:

1. **Sit on the floor with your knees apart and your feet pressed together, soles touching, in the "butterfly" position.**

2. **Lean forward gradually, and you should feel a stretch in your upper thighs.**

3. **Stretch as far as you can comfortably, and hold for a few seconds.**

Having supplies on hand

One of the best things about acupressure and reflexology is that you don't need a lot of supplies and equipment, unless you decide to be trained as a professional. You need just your receiver, yourself, and a few items for comfort. This list outlines what you need to know about those supplies:

✔ **Your hands and body:** Your hands are your primary tools for giving bodywork sessions, but you may also sometimes use your knees and feet. Use whatever works to give the amount of pressure you want. The tools you use for self-healing can be great for saving your hands when working on others, too (see the earlier section "Reaching those difficult places" for more info on these tools).

Keeping it clean

We want to take a moment to stress the importance of good hygiene. Please don't get offended — we're not implying that you're unclean. However, when you're in close contact with another person (and you are when you're performing acupressure or reflexology on someone else), hygiene becomes much more important than it is in normal social situations.

Wash your hands often to reduce the possibility of spreading colds or other illnesses.

Remember that bodywork involves using your hands to treat yourself or someone else. Obviously, this can be tricky (not to mention painful) if you have long, dagger-like fingernails. If you plan to perform bodywork, keep your nails neatly trimmed and at a reasonably short length.

✔ **Mats, towels, blankets, and pillows:** You need a place for your receiver to comfortably lie down. The best place to give an acupressure session is on the ground, using a soft and comfortable mat or pad. Massage tables are great, but you can adapt your session to almost anything. You can give acupressure on a bed, couch, or even sitting in a chair if necessary. The best place to give a reflexology session is sitting in a chair, but you can also give a great session with the person lying down on a massage table or bed. Wherever you decide to give the session, be sure you have a clean set of sheets for your receiver to lie on.

After the receiver is lying or sitting, make sure he's well supported and comfortable. Use rolled-up towels, pillows, or bolsters under his knees, ankles, or abdomen. Keep extra on hand in case you need to support his shoulders and neck, too.

✔ **Maps and charts:** You need maps and charts for a healing session. Chapter 3 walks you through the charts by explaining how they work, what they mean, and how to use them. When you're ready for your session, have your charts on hand to read from and guide your session. Don't worry about where to put them in a session; you can even rest them on your receiver's body while you work.

✔ **Candles, scents, and music:** Although you don't technically need these items, many people like to set a relaxing atmosphere for the session by arranging some candles nearby. This arrangement can provide a soothing, warm setting. Calming scents, such as vanilla, can also help. In addition, some relaxing music can help put both the giver and the receiver in a calm mood. However, you should always consider the receiver's feelings. If he or she prefers not to have any of these elements, remove them without making a fuss.

For optimum benefit, conduct sessions in a quiet area (with the exception of any soothing background music you may choose). Relaxing is tough with lots of loud conversations and other noise nearby. Warmth and ventilation are also important. Achieving the proper balance of warmth and ventilation is tricky when you're establishing the perfect healing session atmosphere. You want the receiver to feel warm (which also helps her to feel relaxed and cozy), but the room should be well ventilated to allow for enough fresh air. You may want to keep a small heater on hand in case any breezes or air conditioners create a chill.

Preparing Yourself to Receive a Healing Session

You may be surprised to discover that you need to prepare yourself to receive a session. After all, you may think that the receiver has the easy part. What's the big deal? You lie down and enjoy! Actually you may need a little more preparation than that. Here are a few tips:

✔ **Don't receive a session with a full stomach.** Wait an hour after eating before receiving any sort of healing session.

✔ **Try to be relaxed and receptive right from the start.** Check your cares and concerns at the door: Don't worry, they'll still be there when you're done, and you can pick them up on your way out — if you still want them, of course.

✔ **If you wear contact lenses, be sure to tell the person giving the session.** He or she will want to avoid any pressure around the eyes.

✔ **If you wear a hearing aid, turn it off so that it doesn't squeal during the session.** Tell your practitioner that you don't hear well, so that he or she knows to speak up when giving you instructions.

✔ **Because acupressure involves stretching, wear loose and comfortable clothing with no tight waistbands or belts.** Also, remove your jewelry, watch, glasses, and other accessories, which can get in the way during the session and also may effect the movement of qi. Although reflexology doesn't have as much movement as acupressure, you'll still want to wear loose clothing for comfort.

The art of being touched

Do you love or hate being touched? You may be a sponge who can't get enough, or you may find touch invasive. Maybe you aren't too happy with your body image, or maybe you have a lot of pain and just don't want to be touched. The truth is that humans are meant to be touched. Infants who aren't touched die. Touch improves well-being and contentment, calms the nervous system, balances regulatory systems, and connects you to the world you live in. However, receiving touch can be a little intimidating, especially with someone you don't know too well or with someone you know very well but not in the capacity of giving and receiving touch. The great thing about acupressure and reflexology is that they provide touch in a safe, gentle, and health-promoting manner.

Here are a few tips for the art of receiving touch during healing sessions:

✔ **Be sure that you're comfortable.** Don't be afraid to speak up if you're cold, the position is uncomfortable, the light is too bright, the room is too stuffy, the scents are too strong, or whatever. This is your session, and being comfortable helps you receive.

✔ **Take the time to get to know your acupressurist or reflexologist.** Even if you're good friends, a healing plan is a new way of being friends and deserves recognition. Talk about any concerns you have, how silly you feel, and what you hope to experience. And then ask your practitioner the same questions. Don't let an unasked question keep you from relaxing during your session.

✓ **Tell your practitioner about the areas where you want special attention and the areas you really don't want touched (or areas that shouldn't be touched because of an injury).** You have the final say over what happens to your body in a session.

✓ **Let yourself relax and enjoy the session** — you deserve a little attention, so let yourself receive it!

Letting your joints be moved

During the course of the session, the practitioner moves your arms and legs to stretch different muscles or to get a better angle for specific points. Don't help! Your job is to relax; every time you help, you actually get in the way. Relaxing and letting someone else move your limbs can be difficult, but with practice, it gets easier. The instinct to help isn't surprising. You were probably a baby the last time someone moved you around. You've worked hard since then to gain control of your limbs, and giving up that control doesn't come easily. But the more control you have, the less you can relax, and relaxation has lots of benefits. Learning to let go of control in a session may help you let go of overcontrolling other parts of your life as well. In any case, what do you have to lose? Just a little control.

Receiving pressure

Some of the points that get worked in a session are tender. A practitioner may apply pressure gently and carefully, but that pressure can still feel a little threatening. Always tell the person working on you if the amount of pressure is hurting you. Most of the time, the pressure feels good, but you can still find yourself tightening up and resisting it. This instinct is usually protective; your body is afraid that the pressure may suddenly be too much, so it tightens to protect itself from injury. The best way to receive pressure is to relax and allow the pressure in. This relaxation permits the person working on you to use less pressure with more result. Check out these tricks for allowing pressure:

✓ Talk to your muscles, instructing them to relax.

✓ Your mind is powerful: Imagine your muscles getting longer and softer.

✓ Visualize tension leaving your body as the pressure comes in.

✓ Breathe! Your breath is the best tool you have for relaxation. When a tender area receives pressure, the natural response is to try to push it out. Instead, try the following exercise:

  • As pressure increases into a tender area, use your breath and mind to release the pressure and the pain.

- As you breathe in, imagine your breath going to the area of pressure. Imagine you're breathing in a calming, healing light. Maybe this light has a color — one that you find calming. As you breathe in, draw this calming, healing color with your breath into the area that's receiving pressure.

- As you breathe out, release your tension and pain, and let the breath carry them out of your body. Maybe your tension has a color. Imagine your exhalation is this color as you release all tension and pain.

Experiencing Qi Flow

Acupressure and reflexology both work by moving and balancing qi (flip to Chapter 1 for an introduction to qi). You can sense and feel the movement of qi in your body. Most people, however, don't pay attention to the subtle changes they feel that indicate energy is moving. Because science can't measure qi yet, some people have a hard time believing that qi really exists. After you receive some bodywork, you'll most likely find that you do notice the sensations associated with moving qi — and you'll certainly feel the benefits.

Feeling qi may be unusual for you, and you may wonder whether what you feel is real. No, you're not crazy; you really can feel this stuff! Knowing what other people feel may help reassure you that your experience is normal.

Acupressure and reflexology are natural healing techniques that have been practiced by people for centuries. They're perfectly safe when performed correctly and with care. Obviously, if the receiver is in pain or has an existing injury, proceeding with caution is important. Start out slowly and gingerly, gradually increasing the pressure while making sure the receiver has no discomfort. If the receiver experiences any additional pain or discomfort, stop the session immediately until a doctor is consulted and gives the okay for the receiver to continue with the sessions.

What you may feel when receiving a session

Receiving acupressure and reflexology is relaxing and fun, whether you're giving to yourself or receiving from another. These healing sessions can relieve muscle aches and pains, but — be prepared — pressure points can be sore, too!

In the following sections are some common sensations people have when receiving a session, but don't expect anything. You may feel all these sensations, some of them, or none of them, and that's okay — bodywork is good for you regardless of what you feel or don't feel.

Common sensations of moving qi

Everyone experiences the movement of qi differently. Here are some common sensations you may expect:

- Tenderness is one of the primary sensations you may feel when receiving acupressure or reflexology. The tenderness usually goes away when the point releases, because the release allows greater flow of qi and promotes greater balance.

- You may feel warmth (or cold) spreading through your body.

- You may have the sensation of an electric current.

- Most people experience a change in consciousness, in which they're both deeply relaxed and highly alert at the same time. This is typical of alpha and theta brain wave states and is considered one of the most important benefits of bodywork. (See the nearby sidebar "It's electric!" for more on brain wave states.)

- One of the most common physical sensations people experience during a session is "the jolt." No one can really explain why this sensation happens, although you can find many theories (see the nearby sidebar for a prominent theory on this effect). The jolt can happen at any point during a session and usually goes something like this: The receiver is feeling deeply relaxed with calming warmth spreading throughout her body. Suddenly, out of nowhere, she experiences a body jolt. The jolt may cause an arm or leg to move suddenly or may cause the whole body to jump. Having a jolt generally indicates that energy is moving through a blocked area. Although startling at first, you may notice that it's also oddly relaxing.

The jolt

In order for a muscle to move, it must receive an electrical/chemical signal from the nervous system. A signal has to obtain a specific amplitude, or strength, to jump-start the circuit. This is called an action potential. Nerve synapses accumulate signals until they reach a high enough amplitude to become an action potential and initiate movement. Muscles can have signals in the nerve synapses that are just under the amount needed to start an action potential. This is called sub-threshold stimuli. Some people think releasing acupoints provides enough additional stimuli to push sub-threshold synapses into an action potential, creating a jolt in the body. After the nerve synapse releases, it can go back to normal, thereby helping to rebalance the nervous system.

✔ In addition to physical sensations, you may feel deep emotions. These emotions may have been locked up in your body for some time, becoming part of the energy imbalance. Feeling deeply emotional is normal, and it's a sign that the session is stimulating strong healing impulses that help to rebalance energy.

The signs of emotional release in a session are crying, shaking, trembling, sighing, yawning, and sweating. Experiencing any of these things during a session is normal. Each sign results in the receiver feeling emotionally more balanced, free, and lighter afterward.

Relaxation

The most universal effect of acupuncture and reflexology is relaxation. Relaxation has many benefits, including the following:

✔ Relaxation allows the body to metabolize and rebalance stress hormones, which relieves stress.

✔ Relaxation lowers blood pressure.

✔ Relaxation reduces muscle tension.

✔ Relaxation promotes mental and emotional well-being.

✔ Relaxation frees the human mind for greater levels of creative thinking, allowing people to see problems from a new perspective.

Sadly, many people don't know how to relax or even what relaxation feels like. If you're one of these people, acupressure will work wonders!

It's electric!

Whenever nerves fire, they give off electricity. In the brain, this activity is measured by an electroencephalogram (EEG). The measurements of an EEG are called brain waves. EEGs measure the four main brain wave emissions — beta, alpha, theta, and delta — and three additional subtypes. Each is associated with a specific range of frequency and type of brain function. Beta brain waves are associated with normal everyday activity; when someone is in beta state, he's awake. Most activities and thinking processes occur during beta state. Alpha brain waves are associated with deep relaxation and alert mental function. The alpha state is often associated with creativity and is useful for stress management. Theta brain wave states are associated with deep internal awareness, dreaming, and deep states of meditation. Delta brain waves are emitted primarily during sleep.

Press here, feel it there

If you're like most people, you expect to feel pressure where someone is pushing. Prepare for a surprise! When you push an acupoint, you're sending energy along the entire meridian. Look at the reflexology and meridian maps in Chapter 3. See all the connections? Don't be surprised when you push a point in your shoulder and feel it in your feet. This is especially true in reflexology, where each point is a reference to a body organ. You may think that you're just rubbing, rolling, and pressing your feet, but you can feel the effect in every organ in your body.

What you may feel when giving a session

When giving an acupressure or reflexology session to another person, you may have big expectations for yourself. You may expect to immediately be able to feel energy. In time, most people can feel the qi moving through the receiver's meridians or collecting in the receiver's acupoints, but you need practice and patience. Try not to be disappointed if you don't feel energy immediately. Take heart: Giving a session can open your awareness to your own energy flow, causing interesting sensations!

An electric current and other common sensations

When you hold two acupoints together, you may feel as if a current is running through your hands and you're connecting a circuit. Although this analogy is useful, strictly speaking, it's not what's happening. Your energy isn't flowing into the recipient, and her energy isn't flowing into you. What you're feeling is a process called *induction*.

The best way to explain this process is with a fluorescent light. Try this experiment: Turn on a fluorescent light and hold another fluorescent light bulb tube in your hand. Bring the light tube near the fluorescent light. You'll notice that the tube begins to emit light even though it isn't connected to electricity! This isn't because electricity has jumped from one lighting tube to the other. Rather, the light tube receiving electricity has started vibrating the fluorescent ions inside the tube. When you bring the second fluorescent tube within the vibrating field, the ions in the second tube begin to vibrate as well. Vibration in one induces vibration in the other when their fields overlap.

The same is true in acupressure. When you feel the electric feeling of energy moving, it isn't someone else's energy moving into you. It's your energy moving in response to the excitement of your energy field. This can work in both directions, and people you're working on may say things like: "Wow! When you touch me I get an electric surge." Remember that they're feeling their own surge sparked by your vibrating field of energy!

Here are some additional sensations you may experience as the giver of acupressure or reflexology:

✔ You may feel hot or cold throughout your whole body.

✔ You may have tingling in your hands.

✔ You may experience the same type of body jolt that the receiver does.

Basically, any sensation you have is normal. The body is simply interpreting energy movement.

A connection with the recipient

When you're giving a session, your body changes too! You may notice that as your recipient relaxes, you relax; as your recipient's brain wave states change, your brain wave states change. This is called *entrainment* and happens when energy fields interact with each other.

Entrainment is a term physicists use to describe the effect that similar frequencies with different rhythms have on each other. For example, when you first put two grandfather clocks in the same room, they each have a similar frequency (one beat per second), but their pendulums are usually swinging in their own rhythms. When you leave them together, eventually they coordinate so that the pendulums are swinging in sync with each other. They have become entrained to each other. This happens to the body rhythms of people, too, including brain wave states.

Usually during the course of a session, as the receiver's energy becomes calmer and flows more evenly, yours does too. This principle works in both directions. If you find the receiver is wired and having trouble relaxing, relax yourself and settle your own energy to help entrain the receiver and promote greater relaxation.

Practice deep breathing and other relaxation techniques to support the quality of presence and effectiveness you bring to a session as the giver. Flip to "Achieving presence," earlier in this chapter, for more info.

Does bad energy exist, and can I catch it?

Negative energy is one of the biggest misconceptions in energy medicine. Is there such a thing as "bad" electricity? Qi is just a form of energy; it's neutral, providing life force to all cells, tissues, and organs in the body. Because qi is meant to move, obstructing its movement creates negative effects. These effects can include a lack of vitality, pain, emotional upset, or any of the other effects we describe in Chapter 1. Unblocking obstructions releases the qi that's being held back, and that relieves the symptoms. So, relax, you can't get what doesn't exist!

Your own imbalance, activated

You can't catch someone else's imbalance, but if you have a similar imbalance, you can activate your own pattern by giving a healing session. In this instance, the principles of induction and entrainment are working when we wish they weren't.

If after giving a session you find that you feel sick or tired or have the symptoms of the person you were working on, you've either activated your own deep patterns of imbalance or you've become overly invested in the session. How do you avoid this?

✔ **Do your own work.** The more aware you are of your own issues, the better you are at giving a good session and the less likely it is that your own imbalances become activated. However, if you find yourself going downhill during a session, take a break. Do some deep breathing and practice grounding and centering skills, which you can find in the section "Achieving presence," earlier in this chapter.

✔ **Remember the principles of Chinese healing.** Who's doing the healing? The receiver, not the giver! If you find yourself taking on the symptoms of the receiver or feeling depleted after sessions, you're overly invested in the outcome. In effect, you're trying to heal the person by taking his symptoms away or giving him your energy. The best way to help someone heal is to stay neutral and let his body do what it needs to do. His job is to do the healing; your job is to offer support.

After the Healing Session

Ideally, the overall healing strategy doesn't stop the minute you stop performing the techniques. For best results, follow up and follow through in the post-session period.

One important part of the follow-up is gauging the receiver's comfort level, especially as it relates to her condition before a healing plan begins. Ideally, she feels better than she did before. If so, and if she isn't sore, she may wish to have another session quickly.

Sometimes, she may feel more pain after a session. This increase in pain can happen for a number of reasons. Maybe you used too much pressure or worked too long in a given area. Ask your friend whether she felt that you were too deep. If she says yes, you'll know better next time. More likely, the person is in more pain because the session woke up an old injury that had never fully healed. You can't heal what's sleeping, so this is actually an opportunity for the healing process to begin.

Chapter 3

The Terrain: Bones, Muscles, Meridians, and Reflex Zones

In This Chapter

▶ Reviewing anatomical fundamentals

▶ Navigating the rivers of life

▶ Charting a path through a session

*A*lthough the ability to heal comes naturally, you get the most out of the experience if you brush up on some basic details first. This chapter provides some advice on preparing for healing sessions. We review the basic anatomical issues involved and give some important pointers on things you need to know before you start practicing your healing plans. After reading this chapter, you're better prepared to get the most out of your healing sessions.

Handling Anatomy Fundamentals

If you read Chapter 1 or already know a thing or two about acupressure and/or reflexology, you know that pressure point therapies are applied to acupoints and reflex points located in meridians and reflex zones. These points aren't strictly anatomical, but finding them is easier when you know a few key landmarks and just a little anatomy terminology. No worries, we aren't testing you!

The first things to remember are the functions of the various body parts. *Bones* form the structure of the body. Movement is allowed to happen because of *joints* between bones. Joint movement is smooth and gliding because *cartilage* lines the ends of the joints. *Tendons* connect muscles to bones, and *ligaments* hold joints together, connecting bones to bones. Most of the acupoints and reflex points you use are located on muscles and tendons, some are on bones, and only very few are on ligaments. Directions for point location refer to nearby bones, or bony landmarks, even though the points are most often located on muscles or tendons — for this reason, we cover the bones first in this section.

On a few places on the body, you shouldn't use deep pressure unless you have advanced professional training. On these places, nerves, blood vessels, or organs are close to the surface and are susceptible to injury. Here's a list of where to avoid deep pressure:

- ✔ **Front of the neck:** Pressure here can signal the body to raise or lower blood pressure. You can also hurt the wind canal as well as different glands.

- ✔ **Armpit:** Although acupoints are located here, you can also find important nerves that can be damaged, so points here should be touched lightly.

- ✔ **Groin:** Nerves, lymph nodes, and blood vessels are close to the surface. Palm pressure (often called *palmar pressure* by healing arts professionals) is best to use here rather than finger pressure.

- ✔ **Back of the knee:** This is the popliteal fossa; nerves and blood supply to the lower leg travel through here without muscular protection. There is an important acupoint here that we use a lot. Be sure to use very light pressure.

- ✔ **Inside of the elbow:** This is the cubital fossa; nerves and blood supply to the lower arm travel through here without muscular protection. There are several points in this area; when you use them, make sure the pressure is light.

- ✔ **Ankles:** You absolutely *must* avoid using many of the acupoints in the ankle region when practicing acupressure on pregnant women (or on yourself if you're pregnant). For more info on this endangerment site, refer to Chapter 17.

Bones: Landmarks in the bodyscape

To locate bony landmarks, you need to look at the full body skeleton, front and back. Figure 3-1 shows you the bones in the whole body. Most of the point locations are referenced to bones and joints, simply because these body parts are easy to identify by feel and are natural landmarks.

Take time to look at the full skeleton in Figure 3-1, and check out the corresponding descriptions of each of the bones and joints in the following sections. Then try to find the landmarks first on yourself and then on as many friends as you can. You may be surprised at how different the landmarks feel on different body types.

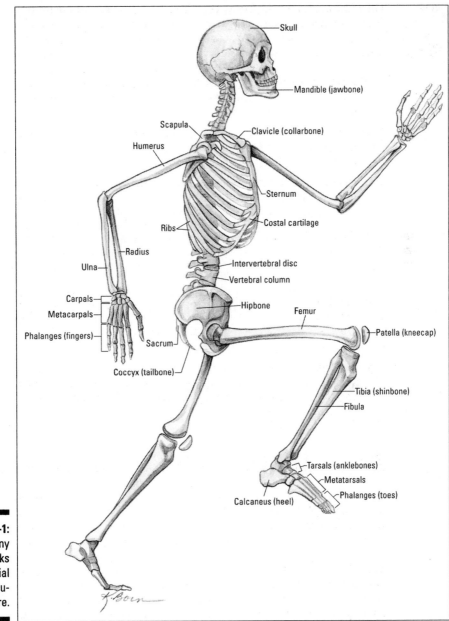

Skull

Mandible (jawbone)

Scapula

Clavicle (collarbone)

Humerus

Sternum

Costal cartilage

Ribs

Radius

Intervertebral disc

Ulna

Vertebral column

Carpals

Hipbone

Metacarpals

Femur

Phalanges (fingers)

Patella (kneecap)

Sacrum

Coccyx (tailbone)

Tibia (shinbone)

Fibula

Tarsals (anklebones)

Metatarsals

Phalanges (toes)

Calcaneus (heel)

Figure 3-1:
Bony
landmarks
are a crucial
part of acu-
pressure.

Although knowing the anatomically correct name for bones and muscles is impressive, you can use just the common names if you aren't an aspiring anatomist. However, you're most likely going to become so excited by the results you get from doing this work that you'll want to do more and more of it. And you may even want to go to a professional training program, so you may enjoy knowing some anatomical names, too. We label the diagrams with common names and we put the anatomical names in parentheses in the descriptions throughout this section.

Anklebones

You use many points around the ankle in acupressure. Reflexology also has organ zones around the ankles, so finding the landmarks here is important. The main landmarks to know in the ankle are

- **The outer anklebone (external malleolus):** This one's easy: run your hand down the outside of your leg until you reach your ankle. Feel the pointy, sharp bone on the side of your ankle? That's your outer anklebone.

- **Outer leg bone (fibula):** This bone runs from the outer ankle to the knee. You just ran your hand along it when you located the outer ankle-bone. This bone has acupoints all along it; press in front and behind this bone from top to bottom and notice how many sore spots there are — each sore area probably corresponds to an acupoint. Acupoints tend to be sore when they're full of stagnant qi. We discuss the concept of qi flow in Chapter 4.

- **Inner anklebone (internal malleolus):** Another easy one. This bone is opposite the outer anklebone. After you find it, use one hand to feel your inner anklebone and your other hand to feel your outer anklebone; compare them. Notice that the inner ankle is slightly higher and closer to your toes than the outer anklebone.

- **Shinbone (tibia):** This bone runs along the front of your leg from the knee to the ankle. It connects to the inner anklebone and ankle.

- **Heel (calcaneous):** The heel is the whole back of your foot. You can cup it in the palm of your hand. The heel has both an inner and outer aspect and both have pressure points on them.

- **Navicular and cuneiform bones:** Sorry, the navicular and cuneiform bones don't have common names, but together they form an important landmark. It's in the arch of your foot; run your hand along the arch of your foot until you reach the highest point. Do you feel a very knobby area? This is where the cuneiform and navicular bones meet. It's more on the side of the arch than the bottom, and it's sometimes sore (as can be the area near/underneath it) when you press it.

✔ **Metatarsal bones:** Again, no common name, but the metatarsals are the five foot bones that lead to the toes. Grasp your foot, and feel the long bones between your toes and your anklebones. Many points run between these bones, so feel the troughs between the bones; grasp two bones that are next to each other and move them, pushing one down while you pull the other up. Go back and forth, loosening the tendons and fascia. Explore all these bones and the way they move.

Knee bones and joints

The knee is another hot spot for good points. The knee points can be hard to locate, so spending time finding the landmarks is worthwhile, making it much easier to find the points during your sessions. Knees are a common source of pain and discomfort, so this is an area that you may want to focus considerable attention on. Important landmarks are

✔ **Kneecap (patella):** The kneecap sits right on top of the knee joint. It's not actually part of the knee joint but floats on top of it in the quadriceps tendon. Straighten your leg and place your hand over the kneecap. You can tell that it's floating in the tendon because you can move it around.

✔ **Knee bump (tibial tuberosity):** This bump, which is on the shinbone, is just below the kneecap and sticks right out. It's the place where the quadriceps tendon attaches to the shinbone, connecting the quadriceps muscle to the bone.

✔ **Outer side of knee (fibular head):** Feel the bones on the outside of the knee. Wriggle your hand down the outside of the joint until you feel the knob that sits at about the same level as the knee bump. This knob is the head of the fibula bone. Press all along it.

✔ **Inner side of knee (tibial head):** Feel the bones on the inner side of the knee. Explore all the bumps, nooks, and crannies where the shinbone meets the femur, or the upper leg bone. Any sore spots? By now you may be getting the idea that acupoints are often sore!

✔ **Back of the knee (popliteal fossa):** This isn't an actual boney landmark, but it's a spot you should be aware of. The back of the knee has two tendons from your hamstring muscles running on the inside and outside of the joint. Right in the center is a soft boggy spot where blood vessels and nerves run. Although good points are located here, never use deep pressure, because you can hurt someone.

Hip, pelvic, and buttock bones

This area is a little sensitive for point location. Some of the points are in, well, personal areas, although we avoid using any *really* personal points. Make sure you show your receivers the locations of the points in these areas before you get started. This way, they won't be surprised and wonder what the heck you're doing. Landmarks for this area are

✔ **Hipbone (ASIS):** The hipbone is the pointy bone on either side of your lower stomach. Put your hands on your hips like you're getting ready to yell at someone, and your fingers fall right on the point of the hipbone.

✔ **Top of the hipbone (iliac crest):** One more time, place your hands on your hips, fingers facing in any direction you want. The bones your hands are resting on are the iliac crests.

✔ **Hip joint (greater trochanter):** Place the palm of one hand over your hipbone, fingers pointing down. Lift your knee up and down. Feel that ball moving under your fingertips on the side of your upper thigh? That's the hip joint. Explore it, pressing all around the contour while moving your leg around.

✔ **Pubic bone:** This bone is the boney plate at the bottom of your abdomen between your hipbones. To easily locate this area in a non-invasive way, place the flat of your hand over the recipient's belly button, thumb toward her head. Press into her stomach, and start moving your hand toward the pubic bone until you hit the boney plate with your baby finger.

The pubic bone is one of the personal places your receiver may want you to avoid using, but it does contain a couple of important points. Just be sure that your receiver knows that you're going to use these points ahead of time and that you both feel comfortable. The way you approach a point is often what makes it sensitive; be firm and definite. Tentative touch makes people wonder what you're thinking about.

✔ **Sacrum:** The sacrum is the upside down triangle at the bottom of your spine. Place your hands on your hips with your fingers facing backward and your thumb facing down. Your fingers reach the edge of your sacrum. If you press around this area, you find a bump on both sides. This bump is the sacroiliac joint. (Note the difference between the sacrum and tailbone [coccyx] — your tailbone is located at the bottom of your sacrum.)

Shoulder blades and vertebrae

The vertebrae are the individual bones of the spinal column. You have lots of acupoints up and down the back, but you probably have a hard time feeling them on yourself. Get a friend and borrow his back for exploration of the following landmarks:

✔ **Vertebrae:** There are 7 vertebrae in the neck, 12 vertebrae in the mid-back (these have ribs attached), and 5 vertebrae in the low back (these have no ribs). Acupoints are beside every vertebra, so feel all along your friend's back and be sure you can tell the difference between vertebrae with a rib attached and vertebrae without a rib attached. It's easy; is there a rib or isn't there?

✔ **Shoulder blade (scapula):** You have two shoulder blades, one on each side of your spinal column, forming the back part of the base where your arms attach to your body. Like the sacrum, they're shaped like upside-down triangles. You should be able to stretch your hand all the way around your friend's shoulder blade (or if you're abnormally flexible, around your own). Find the following areas:

- **Inside border:** The inside border of the shoulder blade is the edge of the blade closest to the spinal column. A lot of muscles attach to the inside border, so of course you can find good points here.

- **Outside border:** The outside border is on the outside edge of the shoulder blade; at the uppermost point, the blade becomes part of the arm joint. Palpate the entire border and explore where it attaches to the arm bone.

- **Superior angle:** This is the sharp point all the way on top of the inside border of the shoulder blade. It really hurts when pressed. You can reach your own by taking your hand and crossing it over to the opposite shoulder. Feel for the sore, pointy spot right at the top of the shoulder.

- **Inferior angle:** This is the bottom point of the triangle, at the lowest part of the shoulder blade. You can try finding the end of the point on yourself, but it's easier to find on someone else. The inferior angle is used a lot as a reference for locating acupoints on the back, so be sure you know where it is so you have an easier time finding those points.

Features of the cranium

The face and head have many landmarks. Because most of them are familiar — like your mouth, eyebrow, or jaw — we don't need to go over them. When you're finding landmarks on the head, be careful not to use too much pressure, because you don't have much padding over those bones. You can find all these landmarks on yourself:

✔ **Cheekbone and arch (maxillary bone, zygomatic bone, and zygomatic arch):** This complex runs from your ear to your nose. Place your fingers in front of your ear and feel the bone. This is the zygomatic arch, which is part of the temporal bone. Follow it to your nose. It starts in a downward direction, turns into the zygomatic bone then curves back up, turning into the maxillary bone toward your nose. The lowest point of this bone, the zygomatic bone, is a smooth knob and is the part we commonly think of as the cheekbone. Acupoints are located all along this complex.

✔ **Eye socket (orbit of the eye):** Place your fingers on your eyebrows. The bone that overhangs the eyes is the orbit. Run your fingers all along this boney socket circling both of your eyes. You'll feel many tender spots, so be gentle!

✔ **Occipital protuberance:** Sorry, this one has no other name. Find the ridge at the back of your head with your hands. Feel the hollow in the bone where the spinal column enters the skull. On either side of the hollow is the bony protuberance (otherwise known as a knob) that you're looking for. Continue to feel the occipital bone all the way over to the ear.

Be careful when applying pressure to this point, because it can be sensitive!

Significant bones of the chest, arms, and hands

We keep the bones in this section to the minimum that are important for point location. As you can see from Figure 3-1, you have quite a few bones here, and familiarizing yourself with them can be overwhelming.

✔ **Chest bone (sternum):** The chest bone is the big bone over your chest. It has three main sections: the top section connects with the collarbones, the middle section runs between the breasts, and the bottom section forms a little pointy knob called the *zyphoid process.* See whether you can feel all these different sections.

✔ **Collarbones (clavicals):** The collarbones are horizontal and travel from the chest bone to the point of the shoulder. They're curved bones that separate your neck from your body. Follow them from end to end.

✔ **Point of the shoulder (acromium processes):** Your collarbones meet your shoulder blades at a point on the top of your shoulder. The shoulder point overhangs the shoulder joint.

✔ **Deltoid tuberosity:** This bump is located on the outside of your arm bone (humerous). It falls just below your deltoid muscle and is tender to the touch.

✔ **Elbow bone (olecranon process):** Okay, everyone knows where the elbow is, right? You also need to locate the crease of the elbow and the inside of the elbow joint. Bend your elbow so that your arm crosses your stomach. See the crease that runs from your elbow bone to the soft inner side? That's the elbow crease. The inside of the elbow joint is another one of the endangerment sites, so be sure to explore this area with care.

✔ **Wrist bone (ulnar tuberosity):** This bone is the bump on the back of your wrist on the same side as your baby finger. It's made by the ulnar bone where it attaches to the wrist bones. Feel all these bones and take your time to explore the many nooks and crannies. Be sure to move the wrist around while you're palpating so that you can feel how the bones all move.

✔ **Metacarpals:** These are the five bones that go from the wrist bones to the fingers — just like the metatarsals go from the anklebones to the toes. Feel the areas between the bones where the tendons run. These areas are important for point location.

Soft tissue: Identifying through feel

Soft tissue refers to connective tissue and muscle. *Connective tissue* is the tissue in the body that provides support to all parts of the body. Although bones aren't soft, they're a type of connective tissue and certainly do provide support. Generally, however, when we speak of connective tissue in reference to soft tissue, we're referring to cartilage, tendons, ligaments, and *fascia,* the latter being the thin layer of tissue that connects all parts of your body, even holding and supporting your blood vessels and nerves as they travel to every cell (we cover it in detail later in this section). Muscle is also soft tissue, and its function (as you well know) is movement. Although muscles and tendons are different tissue types, they aren't totally separate. Muscles turn into tendons as they get nearer to the bones, so the tendons connect the muscles to the bones they move.

The truth is that you don't need to know all the different types of tissue or names of all the muscles. You do need to know the basic layout of muscles, tendons, and ligaments and to be able to feel the differences between them. You need to know that a muscle will yield and accept pressure and that a ligament won't. After all, you don't want to hurt anyone!

Palpating muscles and tendons

Muscles form the majority of the tissue in your body. You need to be able to distinguish between muscles, tendons, and other tissue, but you don't need to know all the origins, insertions, or functions of all the muscles. Knowing the names and locations of the major muscles is helpful simply because we refer to them often. Check out Figures 3-2 and 3-3, which show you the major muscles of the body — front and back — and give you their names. Try to remember where these basic muscles are, or you can just mark this page and refer to it as necessary.

What's important is to be able to feel muscles. Each muscle has three distinct sections:

✔ **Belly:** This part of the muscle contracts the most. In muscle-builders, you can see the belly contract into a round ball when they use the muscle.

✔ **Muscle-tendon junction:** This junction is where the fibers of the muscle begin to interweave with the collagen fibers of the tendons. This part isn't as strong as the tendon and isn't as elastic as the muscle, which makes it the biomechanical weak point of the muscle.

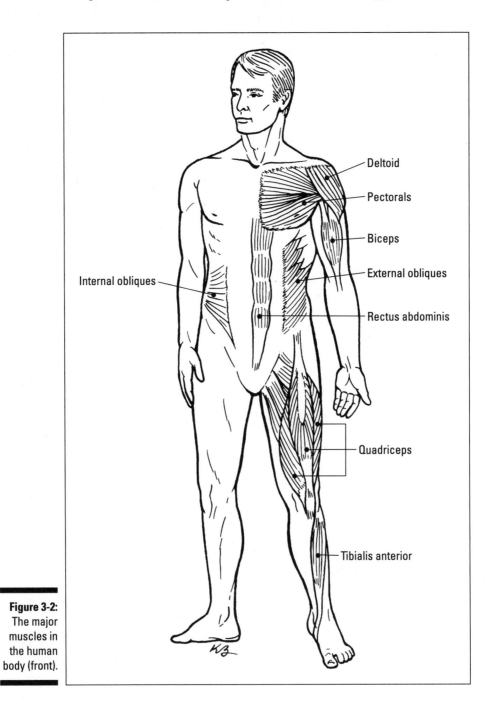

Figure 3-2:
The major
muscles in
the human
body (front).

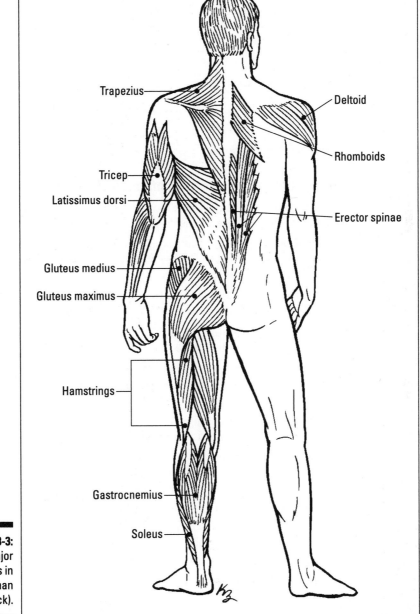

Figure 3-3:
The major muscles in the human body (back).

✔ **Tendon:** This part is the bridge from muscle to bone. Tendons and other connective tissue are made of collagen and elastin fibers — they have a lot of strength, but not as much elasticity as muscles have. As a result, they aren't able to absorb as much pressure as muscles can. Remember this important point when giving sessions so that you don't press too hard on a tendon!

To feel the different sections of muscle and tendon, try this exercise:

1. **Bend your elbow and make a fist, showing off your amazing bicep muscle.**

   No, you're not trying out for a muscle man contest, just picking an easy muscle to feel.

2. **Grab the middle of the muscle — this is the muscle belly.**

3. **Relax slightly by opening your elbow joint just a little bit so that it's easier to take hold of your muscle and move it around.**

   The belly is the thickest part of the muscle and does the most contracting when doing work. It gets thicker and harder when it's contracting, and longer and softer when it's relaxing.

4. **Open and close your elbow a few times to feel the difference between the muscle when it's tense versus when it's relaxed.**

   When you're using pressure point therapy, you want to know whether the muscle you're working is relaxed or tense. Note the following:

   • If the muscle is hard and unyielding (you can't push into it), it's tense, and you need to be careful not to fight with the tissue, trying to force it to relax.

   • If the muscle is hard but yielding, it's a good toned muscle that's relaxed. This muscle can receive a fair amount of pressure comfortably.

   • If the muscle is soft and very yielding, it's a relaxed, untoned muscle, and you need to be careful not to use too much pressure.

5. **See whether you can pull the muscle belly off the underlying bone.**

   Wrap your fingers as far around the muscle as you can. Get a good feel for what muscle tissue feels like. This step helps you recognize how much you can stretch and move a muscle during sessions.

6. **Walk your fingers toward the elbow joint.**

   The muscle gets thinner as you leave the belly; the muscle is starting to turn into tendon — this is called the musculo-tendinous junction. Notice that it's less fibrous, less yielding, and more slippery than muscle tissue. When you reach the elbow there is no more muscle, only tendon. The tendon feels like a hard steel cable and is very strong.

7. Open and close your elbow a few times and feel this tendon popping out.

When you know what to look for, you can easily feel the distinctions between different types of soft tissue. However, every person is just a little different (well, okay, some people may be a lot different), so you may want to palpate a lot of people's tissue to get a sense of how varied it can feel. Be careful, though, and always ask for permission first!

Gently feeling ligaments, the stationary supporters

Some acupoints are located on ligaments, and, unlike muscles and tendons, ligaments aren't designed to move. They're designed for maximum strength to support the joint and keep it from dislocating. As you may expect, they don't have a lot of flexibility and they don't yield when you apply pressure. They feel like slippery strings; they're not as hard as tendons, but feeling the difference between ligaments and tendons can be difficult.

The basic rule of thumb is that anytime you use acupoints near a joint, don't use a lot of pressure. Because the ligaments — and even tendons — don't have a lot of give, nothing absorbs the pressure that you apply. A little pressure can feel great, but just a little more pressure can suddenly feel very painful. This pain isn't the good pain either; this is the "get off my ligament now" pain.

Sliding your hand along fascia

Have you ever taken the skin off a piece of chicken when preparing a recipe? Do you remember the thin, filmy membrane right under the skin and surrounding the muscle? That's *fascia*. It looks like saran wrap and covers every cell in your body; wraps around every muscle, bone, and organ; and covers your entire body underneath your skin in one continuous, uninterrupted sheet! Many people theorize that meridians travel through fascia, and that's why you can feel the effects of meridian therapy so quickly, in so many different places, and on so many different levels.

In a living body, fascia has 2,000 pounds of tensile strength. That means it can withstand forces up to 55 miles an hour before tearing. Pretty impressive, huh? What's really cool is that fascia is more conductive than nerve tissue, so it can transmit an electrical signal faster than a nerve!

Feeling the superficial layers of fascia is easy. Take your hand and place it over your leg or arm without using any pressure — use just the weight of your hand. Let your hand sink into your skin, feeling your muscle or fat layer under your skin. Lift just a little of the pressure from your hand and gently move your skin so that it glides over the muscle or tissue underneath. What's allowing the skin to glide? Fascia!

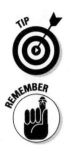

If you're really brave, the next time you prepare chicken, try this skin glide on the chicken. You may be surprised by what you discover.

In the healing plans in this book, you stretch an area before you apply pressure point therapy. The reason you stretch first is to open the fascia so that the flow of qi in the meridian can move better. When you can feel fascia, you have an easier time knowing how much or little to stretch an area.

Meridians: Channeling the Rivers of Life

Meridians are channels that deliver qi to all parts of the body. They're often called rivers of life because qi is vital life energy. If this sounds like Greek, check out Chapter 1.

Understanding meridians and how they work

Because acupressure is wholly based on the qi flow along meridians, you need a solid foundational understanding of meridians in order to appreciate what you're doing in a session. To make the most of your acupressure practice, note the following facts:

- **The human body has 12 organ meridians on each side of the body (24 total), named by the organs they govern.** The meridians on one side are mirror images of the meridians on the other side. Every organ meridian governs the health of the organ it supplies as well as specific areas of the body that may or may not be related to the area where the organ resides. Each meridian also has important psychological and emotional attributes, which we cover in the next section. You can use the organ associations and emotional and psychological attributes to help you decide which acupressure session from this book to provide. We cover this topic more fully in Chapter 4. Figures 3-4 and 3-5 show the organ meridians from the front/side and back views.

Traditional Chinese medicine doesn't refer to the total number of organ meridians (24) — rather, it refers to them as 12 different meridians existing on both sides of the body. Seems like a simple technicality, but you'll come across this number often — so when you read that there are 12 organ meridians, just remember that the reference implies 12 on each side.

✔ **In addition to the 12 organ meridians, two other meridians travel along the midline of the body and are called the *central channel meridians.*** So, it doesn't take a brain surgeon to figure out that the total number of meridians is 26. The two meridians of the central channel don't govern organs but do govern areas of the body and have psychological and emotional associations. The meridian on the front side of the body is called the *Conception Vessel,* and the one on the back is called the *Governing Vessel.*

✔ **Although the organ meridians are referenced as 12 separate channels of energy (the very definition of meridian in the acupressure sense), they aren't separate channels — rather, they're different parts of one long channel.** The string of meridians forms a loop so that the last meridian ends at the beginning of the first meridian. As a result, your qi is always circulating in a big circuit up and down your body.

✔ **The two meridians of the central channel, on the other hand, are separate from the big loop made by the organ meridians.** They form their own small loop traveling from your belly button, down around your torso, up your back, over your head, and down the front of your body, back to your belly button.

✔ **The 12 organ meridians travel up and down the body. Six travel down the back and six travel up the front (with one exception — the stomach meridian — which we tell you about later in this chapter).**

Imagine a river flowing down the back of your body, getting to your feet, going under your feet, and then traveling up the front of your body, making this loop several times. Every time the river changes direction, it gets a new name, but it's the same river. This point is important to understand because it helps you see how a block of qi flow in one meridian can cause a backup into more than just one other meridian. Knowing in what direction the qi is moving helps you to know where qi may be in excess and where it may be deficient. Like a kink in a garden hose, qi builds up on the side leading into the block and is deficient on the side going away from the block. Make sense? Finding the source of the block can sometimes be a challenge, but sit tight — we help you find it in Chapter 4.

✔ **Six of the organ meridians stop or start in the hands, and six of them stop or start in the feet.** To be exact, the hand is the ending place of three yin meridians and the starting place of three yang meridians, while the foot is the starting place of three yin meridians and the ending place of three yang meridians. Not sure what yin and yang meridians are? Read ahead to the next section.

Check out Figures 3-4 and 3-5 to see the meridians on the human body — and if you're dying to know what the abbreviations stand for, head to Table 3-1 in the next section.

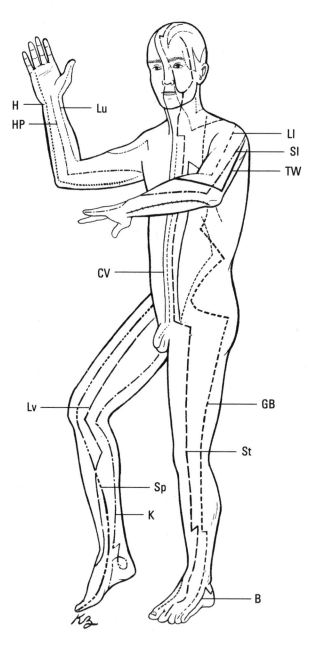

Figure 3-4:
The
meridians
on the
front/side of
the body.

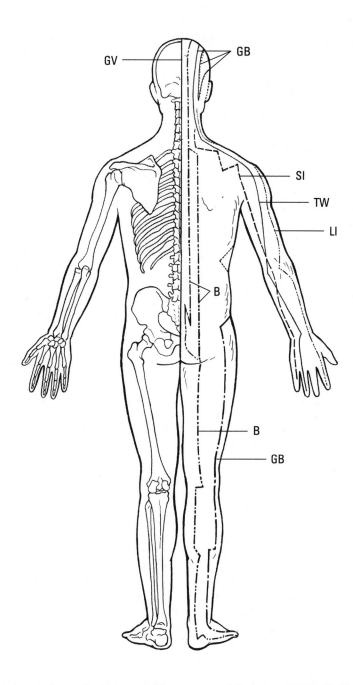

Figure 3-5:
The
meridians
on the back
of the body.

Not only is the direction of qi flow important, but the *quality* of the qi that's being delivered is also a vital part of a person's overall health. Quality relates to the movement of qi: the amount of its vitality, force, speed, and focus. Is it rushing and turbulent, rising to the surface with bounding energy? Is it slow and stagnant, flowing deep inside and difficult to contact? Although blocks in qi are indicators of where emotional or physical trauma is being stored, the quality of qi is often a reflection of the emotional and mental states of the person.

Pairing meridians into yin and yang: The perfect balance

Would you be surprised to learn that half of the meridians are yin meridians and half are yang meridians? Probably not. Would you be surprised to learn that each yang meridian had a yin partner? No? It does seem like a perfect match, doesn't it? (If all you know about yin and yang is that it's a cool-looking black-and-white symbol, you may want to head back to Chapter 1 for a basic introduction to this important symbol of Eastern medicine.)

The division of the yin and yang meridians is simple:

✔ **Yin meridians** are the six meridians that run *up the front* of the body, from the earth (yin) to the heavens (yang). They deal with nurturing, nourishing, generating, and introspection. The soft underbelly of the animal is the yin side, where the internal organs are easily accessible to a predator. Nourishment is derived from the internal organs, and nurturing occurs against this softer underside.

✔ **Yang meridians** are the six meridians that run *down the back* of the body (actually one flows down the front, see the stomach meridian in Table 3-1). They flow from heaven to earth. They deal with defensive energy, protection, strength, and action. This makes sense in a very animalistic sort of way. Think of an animal protecting itself: It takes the blows on its back, protecting the soft underbelly.

Chinese anatomical position is with the hands in a "stick 'em up" position. The fingers are pointed toward heaven and are the endpoint of three of the yin meridians traveling to the hands and the beginning of three of the yang meridians beginning in the hands.

Table 3-1 shows the six pairs of organ meridians plus the central channel pair. It tells you what the partners are, where they go, and the psychological and emotional correlations. The good thing? You don't need to know most of this information to use the healing plans in this book, because we used this info to create the chapters and healing sessions for you to use. The only things you *do* need to know are the names and abbreviations of the organ meridians so that you can follow the healing routine instructions.

Table 3-1	The Yin and Yang Meridian Partners		
Yin Meridian (Abbreviation)	*Yang Meridian (Abbreviation)*	*Psychological Functions*	*Emotions*
Lung (Lu): Starts in the chest and travels down the inside of the arm to end in the thumb.	**Large Intestine (LI):** Starts in the index finger, travels down the outside of the arm, and up the neck to end on the side of the base of the nose.	The lung and large intestine govern what you take in and what you let out. They're involved with making and holding good personal boundaries.	Grief, sadness, loss, low self-esteem
Heart (H): Starts in the armpit and travels down the inside of the arm to the little finger.	**Small Intestine (SI):** Starts on the outside of the little finger and travels on the back of the arm to the outside of the nose.	The heart meridian is "home" to the *shen* or spirit. It deals with personal happiness and listening to your spiritual path. The small intestine takes in, assimilates, and transmits information. If you're having trouble getting the concepts in this book, try using heart and small intestine points!	Joy, over-excitation
Heart Protector (HP): Starts on the side of the rib cage below the armpit, and travels down the inside of the arm to the middle finger. Heart protector has several different names. It can be called Pericardium (Pc), Heart Constrictor (Hc), or Circulation Sex (Cs). Throughout this book, we call it heart protector.	**Triple Warmer (TW):** Starts at the outside of the fourth (ring) finger, travels along the back of the arm, and ends on the outside of the eyebrow. Triple warmer actually has several names, too. It can also be called Triple Burner (TB) or Triple Heater (TH). We use triple warmer throughout this book.	The HP meridian protects the heart energetically because the heart has special importance as the center of the shen. The triple warmer doesn't have a specific organ but governs the three main energy centers that together contain all the vital organs. These areas also represent nerve plexuses in the torso: the brachial plexus, the solar plexus, and the sacral plexus. It governs the overall balance of energy.	Supports joy and protects from overjoy

(continued)

Table 3-1 (continued)

Yin Meridian (Abbreviation)	Yang Meridian (Abbreviation)	Psychological Functions	Emotions
Liver (Lv): Starts at the top of the big toe, travels up the body, and ends at the side of the rib cage.	**Gall Bladder (GB):** Starts at the end of the eyebrow, travels down the side of the body, and ends at the end of the fourth toe. It wraps around the side of the head several times along the way.	The liver deals with planning, decision-making, and organizing. The gall bladder deals with executing the plans of the liver. When your plans are disrupted or obstructed, how do you feel? Angry and depressed! The gall bladder meridian is very involved in headaches.	Depression and anger
Spleen (Sp): Starts on the inside of the big toe, travels on the inside of the leg, and ends at the side of the chest.	**Stomach (St):** Starts at two points — one below the center of the eye and one in the cheekbone — joins together in the jaw, and travels down the front of the body to the end of the second toe. It's the only yang meridian to travel along the front of the body.	The spleen and stomach work together to nourish and care for the body-mind. They're responsible for both physical and emotional nourishment and govern self-care. They also govern mental activity and are involved with clear thought process or too much mental activity.	Worry, concern, reminiscing, nostalgia
Kidney (K): Starts at the sole of the foot, travels along the inside of the leg, and ends at the collarbone.	**Bladder (B):** Starts on the inside corner of the eye, travels down the back on either side of the spine, and ends on the side of the small toe.	The kidney stores energy and the bladder meridian distributes it. They're responsible for the quantity of energy moving through the meridians. They also manage ancestral qi, or carrying out the instructions of our DNA.	Fear and faith

Yin Meridian (Abbreviation)	Yang Meridian (Abbreviation)	Psychological Functions	Emotions
Conception Vessel (CV): Travels between the pubic bone and the collarbone.	**Governing Vessel (GV):** Travels between the nose and the coccyx bone on the sacrum.	The conception vessel and governing vessel deal with your essential personality — who you are as a person. They're important to maintaining the spiritual balance of the meridians.	Centered and grounded

Spotting acupoints along the meridians

In order to fully grasp acupressure techniques, you have to understand what acupoints are and how working with them affects a person's overall health. In Chapter 1, we explain that acupoints are points in the meridian that can be accessed to influence the flow of qi — and the disruption in that flow is what causes imbalance and eventual disease. Here's what you need to know about acupoints:

✔ **Acupoints are closer to the surface of the skin and can be felt more easily than the meridians.** Although meridians aren't anatomical structures that can be dissected out, they're not quite imaginary lines either. With training and practice, you can feel them, and as we discuss in Chapter 1, acupoints may be measurable through skin conductivity.

✔ **Every meridian has a series of acupoints.** The longest meridian, the bladder meridian, has 67 points. The shortest meridian, the heart meridian, has 9 points. There are a total of 357 points in the body (actually, counting "extra points" gives you a few more).

✔ **Every acupoint has its own number and name.** A point is numbered by the meridian it's on and what order it's in. For example, the first point on the bladder meridian is Bladder 1, and so on. A point is named according to its quality. The names are things like "Bubbling Brook" and "Sea of Qi." Don't worry — you don't have to memorize them! We show you the key points for the areas and imbalances that you're working on, and that's all you need to know.

Acupoints balance the meridian they're on, but they also have individual functions. Some of them may stimulate the relaxation of muscles and tendons, and some may influence stamina and well-being. This book chooses points that are specific to the healing plan you're doing. We tell you the number of the point, the name of the point, and the function of the point. We also show you a picture of where the point is and tell you how to locate it. If you've ever played connect the dots, you should have no problem following our instructions and figures.

Charting Your Way through an Acupressure Session

The beginning of this chapter shows you a few bony landmarks, how to feel tissue, and where the meridians are. The next thing you need to know is how to find the points. Fortunately, we have charts that you can use. Unfortunately, the charts are far too complicated for easy navigating. In the healing routine sections, we break down the charts into easy-to-use diagrams for the areas that you're working on, and we use abbreviations to make your reading easier. For now, take a quick look at Figures 3-4 and 3-5, the organ meridians from the front, back, and side.

Distinguishing among the three types of touch points

You've probably heard the term *trigger points* before and are wondering whether they're the same as acupoints or reflex points. The answer is no, they're not. Acupoints are related to energy flow in a meridian and its relationship to organs and organ systems. Reflexology points are related to zone reflexes that influence organs or body areas. Trigger points, on the other hand, are points in a muscle that trigger pain when you press them. They're places where muscle tissue is contracted, and when you press them, they refer pain into other areas of the body. Trigger points can happen anywhere in a muscle where physical trauma has occurred, but they often happen at the weakest biomechanical point of the muscle. Trigger point maps are the places in muscles where trigger points most often occur and show the area where trigger points most often refer pain.

The referral patterns of trigger points sometimes — but not always — follow meridian pathways and sometimes — but not always — follow nerve zones. The most likely explanation for trigger point referral patterns is related to fascia. Fascia is one continuous sheet connecting all parts of the body (see the earlier section "Sliding your hand along fascia" for more info). Fascial strains can transmit the tissue pull from a trigger point to any other part of the body. Here's an interesting correlation between trigger points and acupoints: Although not all acupoints are related to trigger points, 85 percent of all trigger points happen on acupoints. This fact indicates the importance of proper energy flow to muscle function and is another good reason to do pressure point therapy.

The acupoints are located within the meridians, so knowing the basic meridian pathway that you're working on is helpful. Every point is named by the meridian that it's on, so you don't have any trouble knowing where you are. Each meridian name is abbreviated; you can find these abbreviations in Table 3-1, after the meridian name.

The hardest part of understanding the charts we use for an acupressure session is translating a two-dimensional picture onto a three-dimensional body. That's where your bony landmarks come in — see the earlier section "Bones: Landmarks in the bodyscape" for more info. We give directions using landmarks to help make things three-dimensional. From those landmarks, we give you measurements to help you reach the acupoints.

Points on the body are measured differently than points in space. Locating points according to how many inches they are from a landmark is a little difficult. Instead, we use a body measurement called the chon. The *chon* is a Japanese word that means *one thumb-width*. In Chinese acupuncture the word is *cun*. If a point is one chon below the kneecap, you place your thumb against the bottom of the kneecap and the point is on the other side of your thumb — one thumb-width from the kneecap! If a point is two chon from the bottom of the kneecap, you measure your thumb-width twice. Sound easy? It is!

Sometimes a point is so far away from a landmark that it gets hard to count the thumb-widths. Two simple conversions make things a lot easier. In general:

✔ **Two thumb-widths are equal to three finger-widths.** This conversion makes it easy to measure points that are hard to reach with the thumb.

✔ **A palm-width is approximately four thumb-widths.** Go ahead, measure for yourself. Take your thumb and place it width-wise along the side of your palm, with the top of your thumb pointing toward your fingers. How many thumbs does it take to cross the palm? Just a little more than four, usually!

You may have already figured out the problem with this system. Did you notice when you were palpating landmarks how much larger some people are than others? So whose thumb are you using to measure with? A chon is personal to each body. My chon isn't the same as your chon, so using my thumb to measure your body is pointless. I can't very well use your thumb either. Before starting a session on someone else, take your thumb and measure it against your friend's thumb. Is your thumb a little wider or a little narrower? It's your job to adjust each measurement to the same difference. It's not as hard as you think, for one good reason. When you palpate the points as we guide you earlier in this chapter, you notice how tender some of them are. Remember that most acupoints are a little tender; a *lot* tender if the point is blocked up. So when you measure your chon and are adjusting for a size difference, count out your chon and then feel around the area until you find a tender spot. That point will most likely be it!

To practice, we give you a point and a point location, and you try to find it. All you have to do is look at the pathway your point is on, follow the directions to the point you want, and press the point or series of points you need.

Try to find acupoint TW 5. If you refer to Table 3-1, you find that TW stands for Triple Warmer. Look at the meridian maps in Figures 3-4 and 3-5 and you notice that Triple Warmer travels down the middle of the back of the arm. TW 5 is located two chon above the crease of the wrist, with the wrist bent backward — it's between the tendons. To get there, follow these steps:

1. **Make a fist and bend your wrist backward (extension).**

2. **Use your other hand and place your ring finger along the crease.**

   Your index finger falls two chon above the crease. That's good use of the three-finger technique to measure two chon.

3. **Press your thumb between the two tendons (aren't you glad you know what tendons feel like?).**

   Press gently into this point. You found it!

Now practice finding St 36. This point is four chon down from the kneecap and two chon to the outside of the kneecap. St is the stomach meridian. Point 36 is on the outside of the shinbone. Use these steps to find it:

1. **Go to the knee and, using the whole-palm technique, place your index finger along the bottom edge of the kneecap.**

   Your baby finger is four chon below the knee.

2. **Use the three-finger or two-thumb technique to measure two chon to the outside of the shinbone.**

   You're in the tibialis muscle.

3. **Press until you find the tender spot.**

   If you can't find a tender spot, the point may be balanced or numb. Just go the spot you think it is and press. Good job!

Focusing on the Hands and Feet: Reflexology

Acupressure and reflexology have many things in common, especially the belief that energy runs in invisible pathways in your body and is important for maintaining good health. However, reflexology isn't based on the meridian pathways used in acupressure — it's based on zones that the body is divided into, which we explain in this section.

Differentiating reflexology from acupressure

The way reflexology is practiced today was developed in the 1930s by Eunice Ingham, a physical therapist who worked with the system of zone therapy developed by the physician Dr. William H. Fitzgerald in 1917. Dr. Fitzgerald reported that applying pressure to the reflex zone points in the hands and feet not only relieved symptoms but also corrected the underlying cause of the symptoms.

The Ingham Method uses deep, penetrating, and constant pressure on the reflex points of the hand and feet. Many alternative reflexology methods are in use today, and most of them stem from this method. One popular alternative to the Ingham Method is the Universal Method, which was developed in South Africa in the 1980s by Chris Stormer. This method follows the same zones developed by Dr. Fitzgerald but is much gentler, using a softer feel with less force. The way you practice reflexology in this book is somewhere between the two. We teach you to feel the amount of pressure the body can comfortably take when stimulating the reflex points on the hands and feet. This pressure then stimulates the flow of energy to the organs designated by the reflex point.

Although both acupressure and reflexology affect qi flow, the mechanism is very different. In acupressure, you're working directly on the flow of qi in the meridian channel. In reflexology, the flow of qi is being stimulated via the nervous system. Think of it like the circulatory system. Blood flow can be increased mechanically by exercise, massage, or other stimulation; or it can be increased by the nervous system giving instructions to the body to increase pulse rate and dilate blood vessels, which happens when you're excited.

Whether you decide to use one system or the other is often a matter of preference. Different people respond differently and — for no known reason — get better results from one system than the other. Also, you may simply enjoy giving one type of session more than you like giving the other. Many people find that using both techniques together provides the maximum result because it stimulates healing from more than one direction.

Understanding reflex zones

The pathways of energy used in reflexology run in ten longitudinal lines from the top of your head to the soles of your feet (see Figure 3-6). Five of the lines are on the right side and five are on the left, creating bilateral symmetry. Like the leg meridians of acupressure, each pathway in reflexology ends in one of the toes. There are pathways into the hands as well, ending in the fingers. These pathways divide the body into zones. All your organs and body structures fall within one of the zones. The zones end in your feet and hands, where every aspect of your body is reflected in specific reflex points. Unlike acupoints, though, reflex points have no references to bony landmarks.

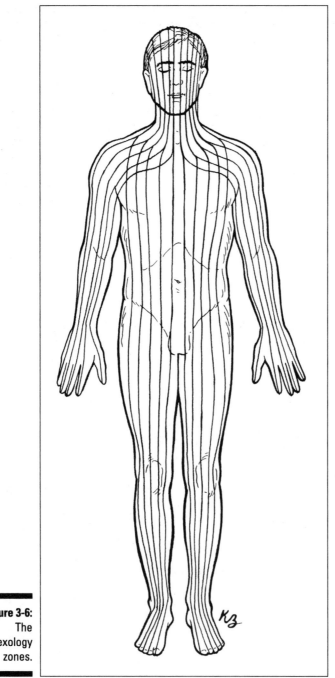

Figure 3-6:
The
reflexology
zones.

The feet and hands are like little holograms of the whole body with every body part, organ, system, and function represented by an area of the foot/hand. Pressing the reflex points can stimulate any part of the body that needs attention. (See Figures 3-7 and 3-8 for the two reflexology maps.)

No one really knows why reflexology works; however, it is thought that the nervous system plays a key role. Although these reflex points aren't directly related to nerve endings, more than 7,000 nerves end in the feet. Before these nerves arrive at the feet, they pass through many tissue, organs, and structures. Stimulating nerve endings sends signals back along the nerve pathways, which may stimulate organ function. These signals may also affect the function of the organs by stimulating circulation into and out of the organs, improving nourishment and waste elimination. So you have many reasons why pressing, rolling, and rubbing the feet and hands can create great health benefits.

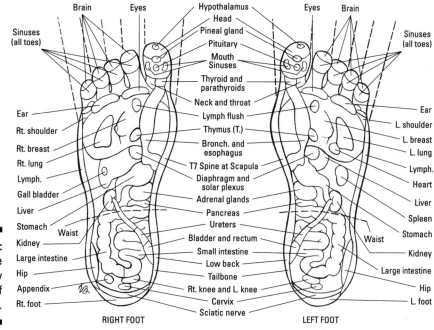

Figure 3-7:
The reflexology map of the feet.

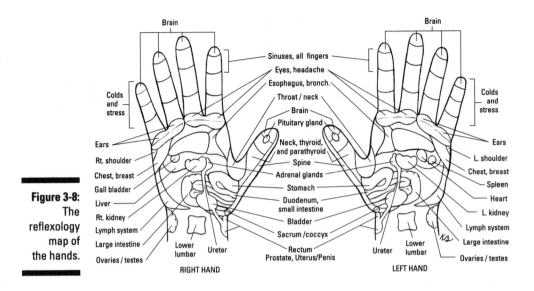

Brain — Brain

Sinuses, all fingers
Eyes, headache
Esophagus, bronch.
Throat / neck
Brain
Pituitary gland

Colds and stress — Colds and stress

Ears — Neck, thyroid, and parathyroid — Ears
Rt. shoulder — Spine — L. shoulder
Chest, breast — Adrenal glands — Chest, breast
Gall bladder — Stomach — Spleen
Liver — Duodenum, small intestine — Heart
Rt. kidney — Bladder — L. kidney
Lymph system — Sacrum /coccyx — Lymph system
Large intestine — Lower lumbar — Ureter — Rectum — Ureter — Lower lumbar — Large intestine
Ovaries / testes — Prostate, Uterus/Penis — Ovaries / testes

RIGHT HAND — LEFT HAND

Figure 3-8:
The reflexology map of the hands.

In this book we give directions for reflexology sessions on the feet. However, any plan we give you can be performed on either the hands or feet. You may want to use the hands when people are ticklish on their feet or don't like to have their feet touched. Using the hands is also convenient when you want to assist someone in a public situation and you don't have the privacy to take off shoes and socks.

You don't need to memorize these maps in order to use reflexology points. You can always refer to charts, even in the middle of a session. In fact, to help you out, we include the maps and legends on the yellow tear-out card at the front of this book so that you can keep it with you at all times (or whenever you'll use it, anyway). It does help, however, if you're a little familiar with the maps and the general organ areas.

Chapter 4

Technique: The Healing Touch

. . . .

In This Chapter

▶ Discovering acupoints and reflex points

▶ Looking at the steps of a healing plan

▶ Examining the beginning and end of a session

▶ Perfecting your healing touch

. . . .

When you understand the fundamentals of the philosophy, anatomy, and therapeutic basics of acupressure and reflexology, you're ready to get into the hands-on practice. As you start your journey, keep in mind that acupressure and reflexology can be easy and effective, but they still require sensitivity and know-how. This chapter teaches you how to find acupoints and reflex points. Then we talk about how to treat the ailments, showing you how to evaluate the problem, prepare the body tissue for the healing session, and use pressure and various techniques to improve qi flow and boost overall health.

Finding What You're Feeling For

Before you begin treating yourself or someone else, you need to fine-tune your sense of touch and know what various textures mean in terms of qi flow. Generally speaking, *acupoints* are small, round areas that can feel "charged," as if you're touching an electric circuit. They function as little relay stations for the qi flow along the meridians. The points generally fall into one of three categories in terms of qi flow:

✔ **They can be functioning normally.** Acupoints that are functioning normally help to maintain an even flow of qi along the line. (Please don't ask how — no one really knows the answer!)

✔ **They can be full.** If an acupoint has excess qi, meaning it's holding too much energy, it's *full.* As you know, meridians can become blocked or imbalanced from injury, overuse, surgery, trauma, or other causes.

When a meridian is blocked, qi builds up behind the block, which makes the acupoints there full, excessive, and overactive.

✔ **They can be empty.** If an acupoint has too little energy (as a result of other acupoints being full), it's *empty.*

Pressing points helps to rebalance them. Pressing full points releases the qi they are holding, moving energy down the line and helping to balance the whole meridian. Pressing empty points helps to fill them with qi and restore normal function. Different types of pressure help to release full points and to fill empty points. We cover those techniques later in this chapter.

Feeling normal, full, and empty points

Throughout this section, we guide you in assessing what you feel at acupoints, so you need to know how to feel one in the first place. Try this acupoint on the large intestine meridian:

1. **Bend the elbow of your left arm so that the thumb is in "thumbs up" position and cross your arm over your stomach. Hold your elbow with your right hand.**

2. **Place your right thumb in the crease of your left elbow all the way to the topside (thumb side) of the crease.**

   You may feel some tendons and muscles — if so, jump over them until you feel the elbow joint, which may put you slightly to the backside of the thumb line.

3. **Explore by using a gentle, circular motion over the bones of the elbow. You'll probably find a very tender spot — that's the acupoint.**

After you locate an acupoint, you can evaluate what lies beneath the surface of your skin.

Recognizing the point under your finger

When you feel different acupoints, pay close attention to what the spots feel like under your thumb, and use these guidelines to determine whether the spot is healthy, empty, or full:

✔ **Normal points:** Usually your finger sinks in when you press normal points and you can feel a bouncy ball in the center.

✔ **Full points (jitsu points):** Full (or *jitsu*) points may feel as if they protrude above the skin line and may feel swollen, warm, and full. If a point has been jitsu for a long time, it may feel hard. These points may be hot or cold, and the ball in the center of the point can feel like a nodule or a little BB. In both cases, when you press, the points usually resist your pressure. It feels like they push back against you when you press them.

Because they're generally overactive, you may have trouble keeping the ball under your finger when you press.

Most of the time acupoints are tender to the receiver when they're touched or even when the person uses the muscle the acupoint is in; other times they're not. The degree of tenderness is related to how easily the qi is flowing through them at any given time, which reflects the overall balance of energy along the meridian. Even in perfectly healthy people, the acupoints work to keep the qi balanced, so full points are often tender on everyone — be careful when you press them!

✔ **Empty points (kyo):** When the acupoints are empty, depleted, or underactive, they're called *kyo* (key-oh). Kyo points are typically located downstream from a blocked (jitsu) point in a meridian. The qi flow is usually reduced, like water in a stream after a dam, and the points on the down side are emptier than normal. (***Remember:*** The direction of flow of the meridians is upward on the front of the body and downward on the back of the body.)

As a rule, kyo points feel depressed rather than protruding. When you press a kyo point, your finger may sink right into it, and the ball will feel deflated, or like it's not there at all. At the other extreme, a kyo point can be so empty that it feels like you fall into a hole and onto a steel plate. The bottom feels hard and impenetrable. This feeling can be likened to reaching the bottom of the riverbed; you have nowhere else to go. When you press the point, it may not hurt the receiver at all and may even be a little numb. But of course it can feel tender, too! This explanation can be confusing for beginners, but remember that a kyo point always feels less active than a jitsu point!

Noticing the change in energy flow

When you hold the points, you feel them change as the energy flow changes:

✔ **When you hold jitsu points,** they may quiver or jump and then suddenly seem to deflate. You may feel the points soften or simply feel calmer. They may have temperature changes and feel less tender to the receiver.

✔ **When you hold kyo points,** you may feel them fill and become bouncier. Or they may start pushing against your finger or suddenly get a charged feeling.

✔ **When you hold healthy points, stop.** Healthy points feel alive with gentle pressure against your finger. They don't really change when you hold them because they don't need to, so you won't feel too much.

After a pressure point changes, move on to another point. You don't need to stay longer because you've done what you were trying to do — effect a change to rebalance the system.

If you can't feel anything, don't worry — it can take years of practice. In the meantime, you'll be quite effective following the instructions and pressing gently. You have enough information from the initial evaluation you do with your receiver to know what healing routine you want to use (more on the evaluation later in this chapter); if you listen to the receiver, she will tell you whether what you're doing is working.

Moving to the extremities: Focusing on reflex points

Just like acupoints, reflexology points in the feet and hands have fullness and emptiness. Typically, when a reflex point is full, the organ it relates to is said to be stagnant or holding energy. When a reflex point is empty, the organ is thought to be depleted and needing energy. When you press reflex points, they can share many of the same properties as acupoints. You may be pushed out of a full point or sucked into an empty point. As you continue pressing various reflex points, you may find bumps, valleys, soft spots, hard spots, and so on. No worries — all those characteristics are normal.

You may also feel something that we can best describe as little crystals that crunch when you press them. Take a foot in your hand and firmly but gently massage it. Do you feel any little crunchy things? Are any areas more sore than others? The crunchy things are thought to be crystallized minerals deposited in your feet because of poor circulation, toxic build-up, or blocked qi. They tend to show up more in your feet than in your hands because the effect of gravity is stronger in your feet, slowing down circulation. Although these crunchy things can sometimes be found in acupoints, they're rare. If you find one or two in your foot, or if you have a few really sore spots, check out the foot map in Chapter 3 to see what organ or body area is being affected.

Don't press these areas too hard — you can cause inflammation. See the section on pressure later in this chapter to find out how much is too much.

Detecting energy imbalance (and balance)

Detecting imbalance is easy! Simply compare one point in the routine you're doing to another point in the routine and decide whether they're the same or different. It they're different, which one is empty and which is full? If you can't tell, ask the receiver. The receiver is the only person who really knows his body, because he's the one who lives in it. You can feel something from the outside and compare it to what you know, making an educated guess, but only the receiver really knows. Press both points with the same amount of pressure and ask whether one is more tender than the other; or ask whether the points feel different, and if so, how. Use the receiver's description of what he feels to decide which is empty and which is full. Later in this section you discover how to balance empty and full points, and every routine in this book will instruct you in how to balance the points.

Walking through the Three Steps of a Healing Plan

If you're starting to think that you'll never be ready to put a whole acupressure or reflexology routine into practice, take heart — feeling overwhelmed is normal. Mastering the techniques takes practice, and the only way to get practice is to jump in, ready or not. Just follow the instructions, listen to your receiver, and don't worry. Whatever you do is bound to help because touch heals!

A reflexology and acupressure healing session has four basic steps:

1. **Evaluate the issue the receiver wants addressed and decide on a healing plan.**

2. **Stretch the area and warm the tissue.**

3. **Apply pressure point therapy.**

4. **Allow the receiver to relax quietly while qi flows through the area.**

   This integration period is a very important part of the session. During this time you may feel warmth, tingling, or a flowing sensation. Allowing for integration helps the qi to more fully rebalance after your session.

Occasionally you may need to skip steps. For example, the receiver may not always have time to relax, or you may treat someone on a bus, pressing points to relieve a headache, and she won't be able to do the stretches. Pressure point therapy will still have a positive impact and is definitely worth doing — it just won't be *maximally* effective.

Occasionally, a receiver feels more soreness after a session or has an aggravation of symptoms. This usually happens when the body is having trouble healing an injury that's becoming a chronic problem. It's often called a *healing crisis* because it initiates healing when the body was "stuck." It almost always resolves within 24 to 36 hours. If it doesn't, a visit to the doctor may be in order.

Evaluation

Before you can embark on a healing plan, you must first evaluate your specific needs and issues and determine which area(s) you need to address. In this section, we give you some pointers on doing this initial evaluation.

What area do you want to apply pressure point therapy to? With acupressure, usually you focus on an area that hurts or has some other symptom. Your receiver gives you this information. You can work where she feels pain, but you probably already realize that where someone hurts isn't always where her problem is. So you may need to play detective and try to find the origin of the problem. Here's how:

1. **Watch how the person moves.**

    a. **Look for stiffness and lack of movement.** If she says her neck hurts, watch how she moves her body. Does she hold one shoulder up higher than the other? Does she turn her head in one direction more easily than the other?

    b. **Look for emptiness and fullness in the body.** Is the chest collapsed and the back overstretched? The person will feel the pain in the stretched area (in this case the back), but the problem may be tight muscles in the chest that pull the back forward.

    c. **Look at the body's relationships of front to back, top to bottom, left to right.** Some people push their chest out and all the attention is on their front; other people collapse their chest, protecting with their back. Does the person you're looking at have a pear shape, heavy on the bottom and fragile on the top? Is she apple shaped, with a big chest and small, narrow hips? Does the person have imbalances side to side? Is one side held higher? Does one side have more developed muscles? All this information helps you decide where the receiver may be holding energy and what areas of the body to work on.

2. **Feel the area where you notice an imbalance to see where the tension is.**

    In general, if you find an empty area and a corresponding full area, you want to use pressure point therapy on both.

The pain in a specific area may be originating from more than one source, so you may need to address several acupoints in order to efficiently resolve the problem. The best way to start is to look at the body, notice the asymmetry, and simply use the person's symptoms to choose a healing plan in this book.

Reflexology evaluation is more straightforward. Have the receiver tell you what issues he has. When you're stretching his feet or hands to prepare them for pressure point therapy, feel the places that relate to different organs. Check for the symptoms that we discuss in the earlier section, "Moving to the extremities: Focusing on reflex points." Work both the reflex areas that your receiver tells you about and what you feel in the foot or hand. You can decide whether you want to use both the foot and hand or only one. Sometimes hands are more accessible, but otherwise the choice comes down to preference. Some people don't like to have their feet touched.

Stretches and warm-ups

In order to get your body in optimum shape for receiving healing, it's a good idea to do a stretching routine first. Stretching helps stimulate the proper flow of energy and increase flexibility. Qi is often bound in muscles and/or restricted by fascia (see Chapter 3 for more info). Stretching or warming up tissue before a session opens the meridians and reflex zones, starting your work for you. Usually you stretch the areas that you're going to work at the beginning of a session. If you're working multiple areas, you may want to stretch an area, do the acupressure or reflexology, and then stretch the next area, and so on.

In this section we tell you about seven main stretches and warm-up techniques — three for acupressure and four for reflexology. You can use one or two at the beginning of each session. Each session plan instructs you on how to do this.

✓ **Muscle stretching:** This common stretching technique requires opening the joint and lengthening the muscles while they're relaxed. Qi flows through tissue, and when muscles are tense and tight, qi flow is restricted. When you're giving yourself a session, you can do simple movements to stretch your muscles and open meridians. We provide these stretches at the start of each session. If you're working on someone else, you can guide him or her through the stretches that we provide, or you can use the stretch in the next bullet.

✓ **Cross-hand fascial stretch:** This technique involves crossing one hand over the other and placing each hand on opposite ends of an area that you want to stretch. Place the hands on the area lightly, with very little downward pressure (see the explanation of fascia in Chapter 3). Then, separate your hands, stretching the fascia underneath (check out Figure 4-1 for a visual aid). Opening the fascia unbinds the muscles and allows qi to flow through the meridians more easily. This technique isn't usually done in self-treatment because it's difficult to do to yourself.

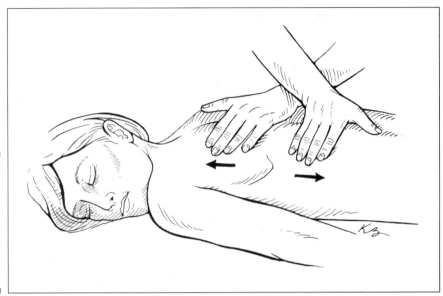

Figure 4-1:
The cross-hand fascial stretch unbinds muscles and encour-ages qi flow.

✔ **Meridian stretching:** As you're working on points, you can do this stretch to help the qi flow through the meridian more easily. Apply pressure to two different points on a meridian using only enough pressure to connect with the fascia. Stretch the points away from each other.

✔ **Foot rolling:** This technique is more of a warm-up than a stretch. If you're working on your own foot, place it in your lap and put your foot between your two hands so that the palms of your hands are on either side of the foot. Gently roll the foot back and forth between your two hands by simultaneously moving your left hand upward and your right downward. Keep reversing this action as you roll the foot. If you're working on a friend, have her sit on a chair or lie down on a mat. Hold her foot in your hands, put your palms on either side of her foot, and roll as you do with self-treatment. See Figure 4-2 for a visual aid.

✔ **Foot stripping:** Place your hands on the inside and outside of the receiver's foot or hand. Place your thumbs together in the centerline of the foot (bottom) or hand (palm). Move your thumbs all the way up the foot and then repeat in a downward direction. Starting at the base of the toes or the base of the fingers, gently and firmly separate your thumbs, pulling them along the surface of the skin. Repeat several times in rows down the foot to the heel and then back up to the toes and also down the hand to the wrist. This technique helps release restrictions in the tissue, which helps release reflex points.

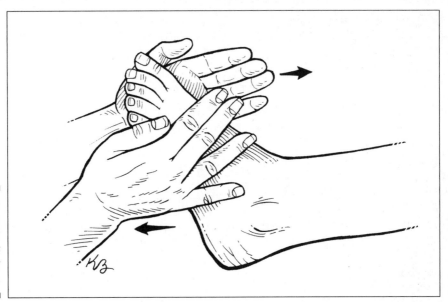

Figure 4-2:
Foot rolling
is a good
warm-up for
reflexology
treatments.

✔ **Finger or thumb walking:** This is a great overall stimulating warm-up for your feet or hands. Start at the big toe, use your fingertips or thumbs, and press and release while "walking" your fingers down the foot and then back up a finger-width at a time (see Figure 4-3). Make a row from your toe to your heel, and then make a row for each toe. This stimulates all the reflex zones. If you're working the hands, start by making a row from your thumb to your wrist, and then make rows for each finger.

✔ **Circular motion:** Use your thumb and compress to the point of resistance. Move your thumb in circles without sliding it along the skin (see Figure 4-4). This is tricky, but you want to move the skin with your thumb instead of moving your thumb over the skin. This technique gives better contact to the tissue under your skin. Generally, you use circular motion all over the foot and hand but especially in the areas that are imbalanced.

Applying correct pressure

In both acupressure and reflexology, pressure is a key ingredient to success. You need enough pressure to contact and connect with the qi, but not so much that you cut off the flow. You also need to know how to position your hands before you even begin pressing, and you need to know how long to hold the touch — this section tells all.

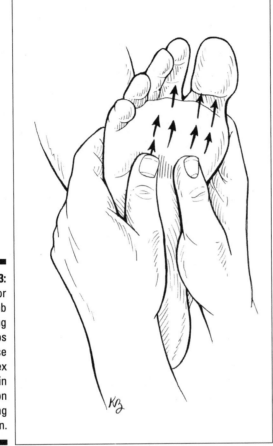

Figure 4-3:
Finger or thumb walking helps release reflex areas in preparation for a healing session.

Where to put your fingers and thumbs

When applying pressure, you can use your fingers, thumbs, knuckles, the heel of your hand, and even your knees! The correct use of your thumbs consists of using your thumb pad(s) to transmit pressure from your body through your thumbs to the acupoint (see Figure 4-5).

You can reinforce your pressure so that you don't hurt yourself. To reinforce fingers, you can use two hands to reinforce each other, or you can use two fingers together on the same hand (see Figure 4-6). Using two hands is especially helpful when reinforcing the thumb.

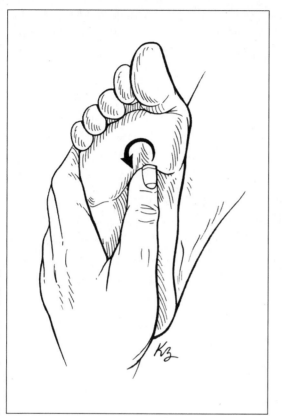

Figure 4-4:
A circular
motion
helps
stimulate
qi flow
where
applied.

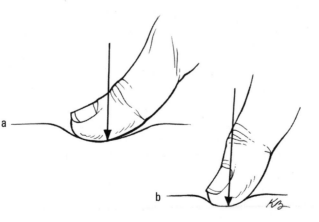

Figure 4-5:
Use correct
thumb
placement
when
applying
acupressure:
a) using
the thumb
pad and
b) using the
thumb tip.

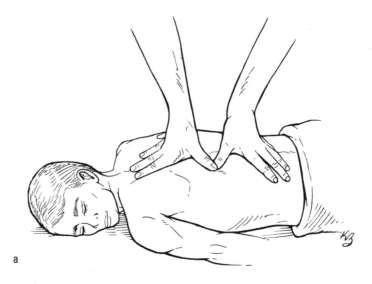

a

Figure 4-6:
Reinforcing
your
pressure-
applying
finger a)
with your
other thumb
or b) with
another
finger is a
helpful
technique
to know.

b

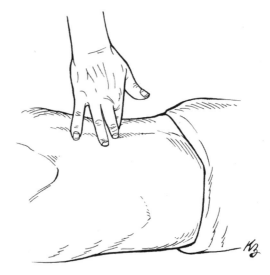

Using an elbow, the side of the heel of the hand, or a knuckle is another great way to give your fingers and thumbs a break (see Figure 4-7).

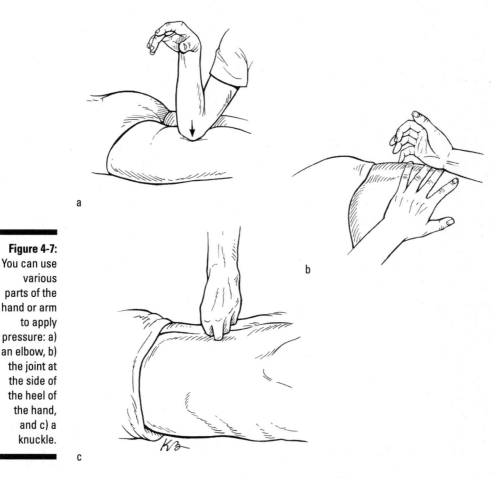

Figure 4-7:
You can use various parts of the hand or arm to apply pressure: a) an elbow, b) the joint at the side of the heel of the hand, and c) a knuckle.

How hard to press

Generally, you want enough pressure for the receiver to feel it. He may say things like "Ah, that hurts so good!" If he says it hurts bad, you're using too much pressure. A good question to ask when you're first starting out is "Does that pressure hurt good or bad?" Asking questions in a way that makes the person choose one thing or another is always helpful. Never ask things like "Is that enough pressure?" or "Is that too much pressure?" People have a hard time admitting that they're uncomfortable, or they may not want to hurt your feelings by suggesting that you're doing it wrong. Let them know that their feedback helps you learn and get better at what you do and also helps you respond to their individual needs.

To know how much pressure to use, you need to listen to your hands as well as to the receiver. When you press into the "ball" of a pressure point, you don't want to crush it; you want to press just enough to compress it. When you feel the ball starting to push back against your thumb or finger, you've reached the resistance of the point. You never want to go deeper than this point; if you do, you'll cause the body to fight your overly aggressive approach. It should feel like it's starting to push back, but it doesn't push you all the way out.

You can apply pressure in a variety of ways to produce different effects. Using different types of pressure is an essential skill, and to do this skill well, you need an ability to find, feel, and evaluate points. This helps you determine how much pressure to use.

Which procedure to use, based on desired effect

You use three main procedures in acupressure sessions, and these three procedures apply to reflexology as well. You use a different procedure when you want a different effect — check out this list for details:

✔ **Work the same points on both sides of the body at the same time (called the bilateral approach — see Figure 4-8).** Imbalances in meridians can happen from one side of the body to the other side. People don't use both sides of their bodies in the same way, and points on one side may be more (or less) full than points on the other, creating disharmony. This procedure is called a bilateral treatment and is commonly used in Shiatsu-type acupressure. To do this type of treatment, press the same points on both sides of the body and decide which side is more full and which is more empty. Then press both points at the same time, applying the techniques to each side as we explain in the later section "Which pressure-application technique to use, based on point quality." This technique can help with left-to-right sided imbalances and is great for overall body harmony, calming frayed nerves, and restoring proper qi flow.

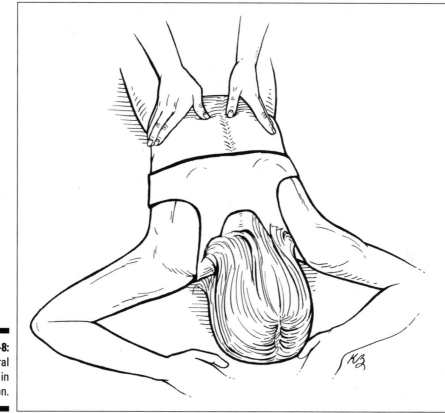

Figure 4-8:
The bilateral approach in action.

✔ **Work points on one meridian at a time.** Another way you can work on side-to-side imbalances is to press key points along an entire meridian from beginning to end, and then repeat the same points on the other side of the body. This approach has the same benefits as working bilaterally but is easier on areas like the arms. To do this, start by pressing and releasing the points at the beginning of the meridian, moving up one point at a time until you reach the end of the meridian. Your goal is to even the flow of qi from beginning to end. You may repeat these steps on one meridian several times before all the points feel even. In general, it isn't practical to press every point on a meridian. It takes too much time and can actually be draining to the receiver to have too many points stimulated at one time. We use this technique in the healing routines and give you the points to balance.

✔ **Balance the full and empty points (see Figure 4-9).** When energy is blocked, you can help by balancing the full and empty points. Balancing the points helps establish normal qi flow through the blocked area. Sometimes balancing the points is enough to remove the block; other times it may help establish more normal flow. Either way, help has arrived. In this approach, you're working different points on the same meridian at the same time. Start by finding the area where the block is. It's usually where the person experiences discomfort, and the acupoints or reflex points here are often tender. These points are your key points, and they're almost always full. Points above and below the block are almost always empty. If you don't know which points to use, try the key points we give you in later chapters for specific ailments. Apply pressure according to our guidance in the "Which pressure-application technique to use, based on point quality" section, later in this chapter.

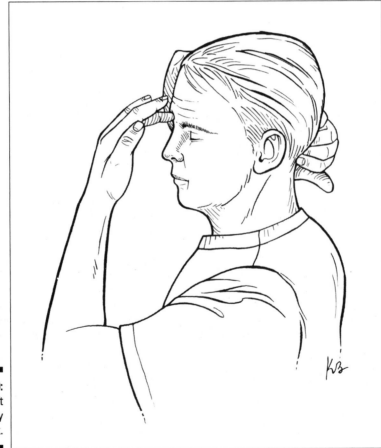

Figure 4-9:
How to shift
an energy
block.

In reflexology terms, you can

✔ Hold the same points on both feet or both hands at the same time.

✔ Alternately press the points selected for the session on one foot, and then press all the same points on the other foot.

✔ Hold different points on the same foot together at the same time.

When you hold different reflex points together on the same foot, you're balancing one reflex area to another. You may want to use this approach when two organs that usually function together, such as the gall bladder and liver, are out of balance with each other. You may decide two organs are out of balance with each other based on what your receiver tells you about his or her problems. To feel this imbalance with your hands takes practice, but you can do it! When out of balance, the qi won't feel *connected.* When they're connected, you'll feel a change in one as you press the other. When they aren't connected, you can press one and you won't feel any change in the other.

Which pressure-application technique to use, based on point quality

When performing a healing routine, the pressure-application technique you need varies depending upon the point(s) involved. Here are some tips:

✔ **When a point is empty,** you want to *tonify,* which means to tone the point or to fill and strengthen it. To do this, use sustained pressure. Apply pressure with your thumb or fingertip to the level of resistance of the point and hold it until it changes (or for 3 to 4 minutes). While holding the point, you can also apply massage in a clockwise circular motion around the point.

✔ **When a point is too full,** use sedating or dispersing techniques. Sink to the level of resistance and then pulse the pressure by alternately holding and releasing the point. This technique helps to disperse or move excess qi. You can also sink to the level of resistance and then massage in a counterclockwise circular fashion around the point.

✔ **To calm the system,** you can use your palms over the points while thinking peaceful, loving thoughts (yes, we're serious). This technique has the advantage of balancing both empty and full points, so you don't have to make any decisions.

How long to hold the pressure

How long you hold the pressure depends on the point to some degree. Every point takes the time it needs to change — and sometimes it may not want to. Your job is to assist the body in maintaining its own balance, so never force the body to make a change. Every tension in the body (or meridian) relates to something that the body is trying to do. For instance, if you have a hurt toe, your body sends qi to the toe to help it get better. You may decide that the toe has too much qi and try to disperse it, but the body always knows best! You can make suggestions to the body through healing sessions, but you can't force change.

Hold a point until you feel it change or release, and then move on. If you hold a point and don't feel a change, move on after 3 to 4 minutes. Sometimes the pressure you apply initiates a change that doesn't complete itself until later. Your receiver may tell you that she didn't feel anything during the session but noticed less pain or tension the next day. Be patient, because you never know what the body may do with what you give it.

You can look for three cardinal signs that a point has released: a pulsation in the point, a change in temperature (gets hotter or colder), or a change in sensation, such as more or usually less tenderness, for the receiver.

Preparing for the Session and Ending It Successfully

Before you can start, you have some preparation to do: You need to get your receiver ready; use the proper props, pillows, and supports; and pick your session protocol. Here's a checklist for putting it all together:

- ✔ **Prepare your supplies:** Get all the supplies you need ready and in one place. Your supplies may include your maps, charts, candles, pillows, and extra blankets, plus any tools you want to use.

- ✔ **Prepare your space:** Be sure it's clean, warm, and inviting. Light candles if you want to, turn off phones, and play music. Place a mat or pad on the floor and cover it with a clean sheet. Have a pillow ready for your receiver's head and a blanket nearby.

- ✔ **Prepare yourself:** Stretch your arms, hands, and whole body before beginning. Practice the grounding and centering exercises in Chapter 1, and be sure that you're calm and focused.

- ✔ **Prepare your individual session:** Before asking your receiver to lie down, take a quick history and see where he wants to focus and what kind of symptoms he has, and then pick the session plan you'll use.

- ✔ **Prepare your receiver:** Ask your receiver to lie down on his stomach or back, depending on the session you're giving, and check to see whether he needs extra supports. If you notice any place where his body doesn't touch the mat, put a towel or support underneath. This extra support ensures maximum relaxation and also protects areas from being overstretched. See the nearby sidebar on props and supports for more info.

- ✔ **Prepare your session protocol:** Use whatever protocol you've decided on, and be sure to stretch the areas before applying pressure.

Props and pillows

Specific areas need to be supported in both the face-up and facedown positions, especially if the receiver has problems or injuries. Although you won't be working on people's injuries, you may be working on other issues they have, and you need to make sure to support the injured area. *Note:* If the receiver experiences discomfort in any of these areas, you should get more material to prop up the joints in question until he or she is comfortable.

Face-up: For general comfort, always place a pillow under your receiver's knees. To ease other common sources of discomfort during treatment in the face-up position, consider the following supports:

- ✔ **Neck problems:** Put a rolled-up hand towel or small pillow under the neck.

- ✔ **Shoulder or elbow injury:** Put towels around the joint to protect it from unwanted movement.

- ✔ **Low back pain:** Put a larger pillow under the knees to open the back.

Facedown: For general comfort, always place a pillow under the receiver's ankles. To ease other common sources of discomfort during treatment in the facedown position, consider the following supports:

- ✔ **Overstretched back or rounded shoulders:** Roll up two hand towels and place them under the receiver's shoulders.

- ✔ **Low back pain:** Place a pillow or folded bath towel under the receiver's abdomen.

- ✔ **Knee discomfort:** Replace the pillow under the receiver's ankles with a larger one.

When you finish the session, be sure to do the following:

- ✔ **Let the receiver relax as long as he wants to.** Be sure that he drinks plenty of water to flush out toxins released in the session.

- ✔ **If your receiver has more pain after the session, ask some questions.** Find out whether the pain is good pain or bad pain. Does it feel like a workout, or does it feel like an injury? Most of the time soreness after a session resolves within a day, and the person feels much better than he did before the session.

Chapter 5

Professional Help Wanted?

· ·

In This Chapter

▶ Knowing whether you should consult a professional

▶ Finding a pro you can trust

▶ Knowing what to expect from the first and subsequent visits

· ·

As we say repeatedly throughout this book, you have the natural ability to heal yourself and others. Still, everyone has limits, and at times you may need to call in a professional (especially if you can't reach the points you need to and don't have a friend who can help). We help you to determine your bodywork needs in the very first section.

If you do decide to see a professional, you want to choose your practitioner carefully. Although a competent, qualified professional can greatly improve your state of well-being, an incompetent one can not only waste your time and money, but also leave you feeling worse than before you started. Or worse, you could end up with a "pretender" who isn't actually a qualified professional at all.

In this chapter, we tell you what you need to know to find your match. Also, because many people are nervous when they first begin receiving healing sessions, in this chapter we help calm your nerves by giving you an idea of what to expect, from scheduling the appointment to experiencing your first session and beyond.

Knowing When to Call in the Pros

Although bodywork techniques are generally easy to learn and can be performed by just about anyone, some cases are best handled by a professional. Examples include the following:

✔ **You or the person you're giving a healing session to has serious pain or is suffering from a long-term injury.** You may need more extensive sessions than you can comfortably perform yourself.

✔ **Despite your best efforts, you're unable to achieve positive results.** Don't be discouraged by this. Some cases can be effectively treated only by an experienced professional.

✔ **You or the person you're giving a healing session to experiences increased pain after a session or finds the session unusually uncomfortable.** This problem may indicate a very stubborn injury that needs the kind of help only a trained professional can provide.

If you're just beginning to study these techniques and are anxious or nervous about your abilities, it may be helpful to receive (or observe) one or two sessions in order to become more familiar with any specific aspects that concern you.

Perusing Your Options

Under the broad umbrella of healing-arts professionals are several specialties from which you can choose your particular acupressure or reflexology provider. They include the following folks:

✔ **Reflexologists:** As you can guess from the name, reflexologists specialize in performing reflexology techniques. Depending on the state they're located in, they may need to meet certain licensing requirements (more on that topic later in this chapter).

✔ **Acupressurists:** Again, this one is a no-brainer. These types of professionals specialize in acupressure techniques. Licensing requirements vary.

✔ **Massage therapists and other professionals:** Some professional providers refer to themselves by other titles but are trained in the art of acupressure and/or reflexology. Look for massage therapists or holistic healers who mention bodywork or ancient Chinese medicine in their ads. Some massage professionals are trained in both reflexology and acupressure techniques, which allows you to enjoy the best of both worlds.

✔ **Acupuncturists:** Generally acupuncturists don't perform acupressure because it requires separate training in finger pressure technique and, more importantly, takes more time to perform. However, some do, so check the promotional material and credentials of the acupuncturist you're interested in.

✔ **Pedicurists:** Pedicurists often take additional training in reflexology as an adjunct to their work. Receiving reflexology in this setting is primarily for relaxation and stress reduction.

Looking in All the Right Places

So you're ready to try to find a healing practitioner, but you're not sure where to look. Here are some suggestions:

- ✔ **The Yellow Pages:** When you're searching for a bodywork practitioner, the phone book is as good a place to start as any. Look under reflexology or acupressure first, and if you have no luck there, try the more general category for massage or acupuncture.

  Beware of phone directory listings or classified ads for "massage" providers that sound at all suspicious or questionable. These are often just thinly disguised ads for escort services.

- ✔ **Online directories:** Many reflexology and acupressure organizations and Web sites have a list of resources, which often includes a directory of providers. On online acupressure/reflexology groups and message boards, users often post recommendations of good practitioners (and warnings about not-so-good ones). Check out the appendix for the organizations' contact information.

- ✔ **Tips from like-minded individuals:** When you're looking for a practitioner, ask around at health-food stores, yoga centers, and other places where people who practice a holistic, natural lifestyle tend to gather.

- ✔ **Word-of-mouth referrals:** As with any other type of professional or service provider, often the best way to find a good candidate is through word-of-mouth. Ask your friends, relatives, and neighbors for the names of any practitioners they used with positive results.

Separating the Quacks from the Pros

Unfortunately, massage therapy (and the specialties that fall under that general umbrella) tends to attract a small segment of less-than-qualified "practitioners." Because of loose licensing/qualification requirements in some areas, almost anyone can hang up a sign claiming to be a "specialist." Legitimate massage therapists don't refer to themselves as "masseuse" and are quite offended if you do. *Masseuse* and *escort* are often code words offering more services than you may be intending.

In order to avoid being fleeced by one of these quacks, check out the info in the following sections and rely on your own common sense and intuition.

Being knowledgeable and inquisitive about licensing and certification

The specific licensing/certification requirements governing bodywork practitioners vary from place to place. Frequently, these professionals are licensed or certified in another area of healthcare or treatment, such as massage therapy or chiropractic care.

Licensing and certification is kind of a tricky area, because as you go from place to place, the healing arts are seen in different ways in the eyes of the law. Some states have a so-called "massage law" governing the licensing of massage and bodywork practitioners — these laws require that any person charging money for healing sessions that include touching the body and manipulating tissue must have a massage license from an accredited school with a specified training program. This includes acupressure, because you manipulate tissue when you stretch it. You'd think it would also include reflexology, but it often doesn't, because it's been overlooked. Other states don't have such laws, so anyone can practice as a professional even after only reading a book or taking a weekend course. And in still other states, a massage law exists, but reflexology is exempt from it. Only a couple of states have legislation that specifically covers reflexology, because it isn't universally recognized as a valid modality. Public education on the benefits of reflexology and its scientific validity are greatly needed.

Contact the health department or the department of education in your local municipality to find the rules that apply in your area.

Doing some background research

These days, the Internet makes it pretty easy to get the scoop on just about anyone. After you find a practitioner who you think may be a good match for you, do your research and check out the person's background and reputation. Cover your ground with the following steps:

1. **Check the professional organizations that govern the modality you're interested in.**

   They usually have a member board of licensed professionals, and they also provide a list of practitioners who have been censored by the organization. We list these organizations in the appendix.

2. **Check the accreditation boards for the modality you're interested in to find out whether the school your practitioner went to is accredited.**

   You can find reflexology and acupressure accreditation organizations in the appendix.

3. **Contact your local training centers and ask for direct referrals of students from the school.**

   You can also inquire as to the credentials of the practitioner you're interested in.

4. **Check the Better Business Bureau and other consumer protection groups to make sure that this person or facility has received no complaints.**

5. **Check for online referral boards that give personal references from people who have used the service you're interested in; in this case, acupressure or reflexology.**

Getting to know your prospective practitioners

When evaluating potential practitioner candidates, don't be reluctant to ask questions. Good professionals understand that this is a big decision for you, and they're happy to answer whatever questions you may have. They want to put your mind at ease and make sure you're totally comfortable that you're making the right choice.

So, what exactly should you ask? Some of your questions depend on your specific circumstances, but, in general, you want to find out about the practitioner's background and training. You also want to get an idea of what a typical session is like.

Here are a few basic questions that you may want to ask:

✔ Where did you get your acupressure and/or reflexology training?

✔ What were the requirements in order to earn the certificate or graduate from the program? Accredited training programs give certificates that most people display. Licensed states require that the state license be prominently displayed for consumer protection. Look for both.

   Fortunately, spotting unqualified pretenders is usually pretty easy. Most likely, they won't be able to prove that they've had any formal training or education.

✔ How much experience in the field do you have?

✔ What is your overall philosophy of healing?

✔ What can I expect from a typical session?

✔ How much will the session cost? What is your cancellation policy?

Also, try to find out as much as you can about the practitioner's philosophy on and attitude toward healing and well-being. These views are very individual and vary greatly from one person to another. No answers are necessarily right or wrong here — you mainly want to make sure the practitioner's ideas are in sync with your own.

You also want to be in sync with the practitioner's level of professionalism. Lack of professional demeanor or facilities can be a big red flag. Mostly, though, you should rely on your sixth sense. If your instinct is telling you that something isn't right, just keep on walking and look for another candidate.

This process isn't a one-way street. The practitioner should also be asking you some questions about what you're looking for in a practitioner, and what your long-term goals are — in other words, what you ultimately hope to get out of this treatment. In some cases, the practitioner may realize that he or she can't meet your needs, or that the two of you may not be the perfect match. In that case, the practitioner should be honest and upfront with you. Don't take this personally — be thankful for the practitioner's honesty and continue with your search.

Preparing for Your First Visit

Now it's time for the actual visit, and at this point you may be starting to get nervous. You may feel silly seeking this kind of help, wondering about its legitimacy and effectiveness. Maybe you feel concerned about being touched, especially if you're not so happy about or comfortable with your body. Or perhaps you're concerned that the treatment will be painful or uncomfortable. Some people, and this may be you, are afraid they'll do something embarrassing, like pass gas, burp, or fall asleep.

Relax. This type of session meets you right where you are, sans judgment or embarrassment. The goal of healing therapy is to fix anything that's out of whack with your energy flow and to right any imbalances. Bottom line: You'll almost surely feel better, perhaps even like a new person.

So, here's how to prepare for your first appointment:

1. **Make the appointment.** Obviously, this task is simple, but you should give it a little thought. Choose the timing of your first visit carefully. You want to be able to concentrate fully on everything the practitioner says and does, so you should schedule this appointment for a day when your schedule is relatively light and when you can relax afterward. You don't want to be distracted because you're worried about rushing off to someplace else.

This initial visit is generally more time-consuming than the average session. Generally, you should plan on spending about 1½ hours for your first appointment. Later appointments typically are about an hour long, but they vary, based on your specific needs.

When you make the initial appointment, be sure to ask whether you need to bring anything with you, such as a list of your questions and concerns. The more prepared you are, the more smoothly and efficiently that first visit will go and the better the healing plan you can put in place.

2. **Prepare yourself mentally.** If you're skeptical, nervous, or tense, your mood will affect your qi flow. (For more information on how your thoughts and emotions affect your qi, head to Chapters 7 and 8.) However, bodywork modalities meet you where you are, and if you come into the session with a closed mind, your practitioner will focus on expanding it during the session. The result? You may have a more open mind when you leave, but if you're going for help with a specific ache or pain, make that the focus of the session by arriving with an open mind!

You may need to give yourself a little attitude adjustment, especially if you're new to the world of holistic medicine and ancient healing therapies. Acupressure and reflexology don't fit the preconceived mold that many people may put healing therapies in (when envisioning "healing," people often picture a sterile impersonal environment like a doctor's office with many pieces of medical equipment around). Because bodywork is derived from ancient healing practices, as opposed to "conventional" medicine, it may seem a bit foreign at first.

Your First Appointment

So, it's time for your first appointment. In the following sections, we give you a general overview of what to expect.

The initial examination

During your first visit, the practitioner conducts an initial examination. This session usually takes a little longer than a regular session because the practitioner has a lot of information to collect.

This initial examination for acupressure involves what are called the *four assessments*. Although not verbally formalized, reflexology uses these same four tools, but not to the same degree of detail. To find out where your energy imbalance is, your practitioner does the following, in this order:

1. **Looks:** Your practitioner begins looking as soon as you walk in the room, assessing how you move to identify places where qi isn't flowing or seems to be in excess: What is stiff, what is free, how your arms swing, and what your gait is like. What else does the practitioner look for? She may take note of your body language, watching how you present yourself and especially checking out your general expression of vitality. Are you full of energy, vivacious, and present in conversation? Or are you tired, mentally unfocused, and lacking connection in your conversation with your practitioner?

   You may be surprised to learn that the practitioner may be interested in the colors you're wearing, your clothes, and your accessories. This interest isn't a fashion critique; the practitioner is interested because colors are related to specific meridians. If you always wear a certain color or always avoid a certain color, it can tell your practitioner which meridians may be unbalanced or overused. (See the nearby sidebar "Meridian color associations" for more information.)

2. **Listens:** Your practitioner uses listening skills as well. She listens to what you have to say — such as any comments you make about what hurts — but also listens to what you *don't* say, which can be just as revealing. You may avoid talking about what you don't want to see or think about, which can be addressed in the session. An attentive practitioner can learn a lot by paying attention to what you don't like to talk about. She assesses the quality of your voice, listening to the strength, force, and tension. This tells about the strength of your qi and how much emotional tension you may be carrying. The same words can be expressed in a lot of ways.

3. **Asks:** During the course of the interview, the practitioner delves into the issues you want help with. She will ask all the regular questions, such as past medical history, medications, family history, stress, relationships, work load, and so on. Then she may ask a lot of questions that may initially seem strange: what you eat, what your routines are like, how much sleep you get, how well you sleep, and whether you feel rested when you get up. She asks you about exercise, fitness, and fatigue levels — generally, about how healthy your lifestyle is.

   Contrary to what you may think, your practitioner isn't trying to kill time by engaging in a lot of small talk. Each meridian has heightened function at certain times of day and in certain seasons. If you always have an energy drop at the same time, or prefer a certain season, these are indicators of meridian imbalance.

4. **Palpates:** Finally, based on the information that has been gathered, your practitioner may spend about 10 minutes palpating key points on the meridians that indicate the overall balance of the entire meridian. The practitioner notes any sore areas, empty or full points, and asymmetries, and she uses that information later in the session. If your bodywork practitioner notices any serious medical conditions that are cause for concern (which does indeed happen), she may suggest that you see an appropriate medical specialist.

Acupressurists and reflexologists aren't trained doctors, so don't rely on them to find medical conditions; check out any concerns you have with your primary-care physician.

These four assessments involve much more than just your physical complaint; they encompass many areas of daily life. Signs and symptoms are a good place to start, but finding the area of imbalance takes perception and time.

Practitioners of Chinese medicine use all the information gathered through the assessment tools to discover a person's "pattern of disharmony." This pattern is based on a constellation of all the signs and symptoms that have been organized for thousands of years into treatable categories. This is partly why practitioners ask so many questions; they're gathering up the necessary components needed to pinpoint this pattern. This holistic approach takes the specific disorder or problem into context within both the body-mind and the total person in whom the condition exists. As a result, this approach is very individualistic and timely.

Discussing your goals and creating a healing plan

During the initial visit, your practitioner spends some time discussing your goals and finding out what you hope to get out of the session. To some extent, these goals may be easy to identify. If you've been experiencing chronic back pain, for example, your initial goal is to alleviate some of that pain.

You also want to mull over some broader, long-term goals. If you've been plagued by repeated cases of the flu or other chronic conditions, you may hope to give your immune system a boost so as to reduce these incidents. Or perhaps you want to be able to do things that are currently off limits due to pain, and you hope to get to a point where you need only occasional mainte-nance visits. (To address the problems fully, of course, you need to rebalance the conditions in your life that caused the problem to begin with. This means that you need a commitment to explore how your thoughts, attitudes, and emotions help to create imbalances that express themselves physically. For more information, consult Chapters 7 and 8.)

It's important not to limit your goals to the physical. Perhaps you also hope to achieve more balance in your life or to reduce stress (or at least find a way to deal better with the stress you can't avoid). You may be a little chal-lenged to pinpoint these issues, put them in words, and then use those words as a springboard to come up with an appropriate course of therapy, but the effort is worth it, because these issues can respond well to bodywork ses-sions. And, as you've probably realized by now, the body and mind go hand in hand: After you address any spiritual or emotional issues you may be facing, it's almost inevitable that you'll begin to feel much better physically.

Meridian color associations

In ancient Chinese medicine, color was considered to be important in relation to the various parts of the body and how those parts were functioning. In five-element theory, a practice within Chinese medicine, each set of meridian partners is related to an element and has a color association. The elements of Chinese medicine aren't the same elements that you're probably used to. Here are the elements, meridians, and their colors:

Element	Meridians	Color(s)
Earth	Stomach and Spleen	Yellow
Metal	Lung and Large Intestine	White
Water	Kidney and Bladder	Black/Blue
Wood	Liver and Gall Bladder	Green
Fire	Heart and Small Intestine; Heart Protector and Triple Warmer	Red

This visit is no time to be shy, so speak up! The more open and honest you are with the practitioner, the better he can guide you in figuring out the best plan of action for your needs and issues.

Together, you and your practitioner will formulate a healing plan, which will vary widely depending on your particular goals and needs. After you have your healing plan, the practitioner can suggest specific steps toward reaching your goals.

If you have several areas that are causing you pain, for example, the practitioner may suggest a healing plan that includes more frequent sessions and specific targets in each session. He may suggest that you come once or twice a week depending on the severity of the issue. Someone who is seeking preventive care may need less-frequent visits focused more on well-being and stress reduction. This person may have a session only once a month.

The frequency of healing sessions is ultimately your decision. It depends on many factors, such as how helpful you feel the sessions are, what other modalities you are using, and of course your financial situation. For the majority of people, insurance doesn't cover these sessions. Consequently, your finances, not to mention time, will be a driving factor. Be assured that whatever the level of commitment you can make, you'll still benefit from the healing sessions.

Some insurance companies do cover "massage modalities," which can include acupressure and reflexology, if one has been prescribed by a doctor and/or relates to an auto accident.

Keep your expectations realistic. If you've been having back pain for ten years, it's unrealistic to expect the pain to disappear overnight, even with the best sessions. Focus on tiny steps and small goals, and you're more likely to enjoy successful results.

Finally, the healing session

Now that you have all the talking and planning out of the way, it's time to get down to the real heart of the appointment: your healing session. Many practitioners like to do a short hands-on session in the first visit after the intake; others do the intake and schedule a second appointment for the hands-on session. Some practitioners charge more for the initial visit, and others charge the same amount as a regular hands-on session. Some practitioners shorten the whole intake, just focusing on your chief goal and not tailoring the session beyond that. This wide variety can cause a lot of confusion, so ask your potential practitioner how he handles it before you commit to a session.

You may be so eager to reach this point that you'll feel like jumping for joy when it has finally arrived. Here's what to expect:

1. **If you're having an acupressure session, you lie on a massage table or shiatsu mat. You stay fully clothed, but loose clothing is best to make stretching easier. If you're having a reflexology session, you take a seat, fully clothed (minus socks and shoes), in a reflexology chair.**

   The room will have low lighting, may have aromatherapy scents, and will be warm and comfortable. It isn't possible to eliminate all distractions, like building or traffic noises, but as the session progresses, you won't even notice them.

2. **Your healing session begins, and the practitioner performs the techniques outlined in Chapter 4 on the points that need to be balanced.**

   The session usually lasts an hour.

   The practitioner may talk to you during the session, giving observations or asking questions, depending on your session goals. If you prefer quiet, you can say so.

   If you were nervous about this treatment, you may discover that you got yourself all worked up needlessly. Most likely, you'll find yourself quickly becoming relaxed as your practitioner begins performing soothing techniques that may result in noticeable improvements in your stress level and in any pain or discomfort that you may have been experiencing.

3. **After the session, you get a few minutes to relax before you have to get up.**

4. **The practitioner tells you any pertinent findings and makes self-care suggestions, and then you book another session.**

In your follow-up sessions, some issues will get better, revealing other issues underneath. Like peeling an onion, you can always work on something underneath. Each session will contain a re-evaluation of the issues and goals, so expect to spend about 10 minutes at the start of every follow-up session re-assessing. How long you continue will depend on results. You may notice steady improvement and want to stay focused on weekly sessions. You may feel so good that you want to schedule a monthly tune-up, or it may not be helping and you may decide to stop. In all cases, your practitioner can help guide the decision-making process.

Part II

Promoting Emotional and Physical Wellness

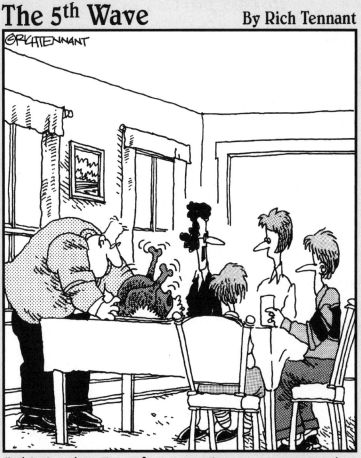

"This is what I get for marrying an acupressurist. Every Thanksgiving he's got to monitor the turkey's Qi flow before he'll carve it."

In this part . . .

You can't have physical wellness unless you also have emotional balance and harmony. This issue is so important that we devote this part to the relationship between physical and emotional health.

We cover the importance of regular maintenance, and we teach you how to monitor — and react to — changes in your qi. We also include some routines to help prevent future problems. In addition, we go into detail about yin and yang, and the process by which emotions are stored in the body, thus causing physical problems. We then share techniques for handling (and avoiding) anxiety, stress, depression, and other factors that threaten your emotional health. To sum it up, this part tells you everything you need to know about the crucial body-mind connection and how it impacts the healing process.

Chapter 6

Maintaining Good Health

*W*hen you think about it, most people take steps in their everyday lives to preserve their good health (assuming they're lucky enough to enjoy good health). For example, most people brush their teeth several times a day without even giving it a second thought, but it's perhaps the most important thing that they can do to protect their dental health. Then there are other, smaller steps that can make a big difference to overall health. Some people take a daily dose of Vitamin C to try to keep colds at bay, while many others make a multivitamin part of their daily routine.

Now you can add one more thing to this arsenal against illness: therapeutic healing plans. Even if you're lucky enough not to have discomfort from any injuries or illnesses right at this moment, bodywork can still help you. By encouraging spiritual and physical balance and harmony, and allowing the proper flow of energy, healing therapy can prevent the energy imbalances and roadblocks that contribute to some sources of pain. In this chapter, we discuss the various ways that acupressure and reflexology can help you maintain your good health — and what you can do to encourage this process.

The Importance of Regular Maintenance (And How Healing Plans Can Help)

As any health professional can tell you — and as most people already know — regular maintenance is important for optimal health. Be diligent about this maintenance for all facets of your health: physical, mental, and emotional. Optimal wellness is expressed not only by a lack of sickness or symptoms, but also by vitality, motivation, and general well-being.

Keeping all your systems on an even keel — and maintaining optimum energy levels and a balanced state — makes your body better equipped to fight off any imbalances, and to heal from any injuries it may sustain. Maintaining the natural balance of vital life forces is important in keeping your system strong enough to handle whatever may come your way. And acupressure and reflexology can take you well on your way to doing just that, primarily in two overarching areas: emotional stability and overall energy flow. In particular, these healing arts help maintain wellness by strengthening qi and balancing the yin and yang forces in the body.

Nurturing emotional strength and stability

Enjoying good physical health is difficult — perhaps even impossible — when you don't have emotional balance and well-being. Sooner or later your unstable emotional state has an impact on how you feel physically. Disruptions in your emotional balance almost always trigger physical symptoms. When you feel worried or scared, you automatically have a physical reaction — tension in your shoulders, perhaps, or clenching your hands and fingers. Needless to say, this wreaks havoc with your physical health and well-being.

Emotional stress can also trigger unhealthy reactions that can have a negative effect on your long-term physical health. For example, when you're stressed or worried, you may eat too much, smoke cigarettes, or drink excessive amounts of alcohol. You may also have trouble sleeping. These reactions set off an unhealthy downward spiral, because your declining physical state increases your emotional stress.

In addition, when your emotional state is unbalanced — because you're worried, stressed, angry, or upset, for example — your body must use precious energy and resources to try to deal with that situation. Meanwhile, it has fewer available resources to handle other crises, leaving you more vulnerable to illness and other physical problems.

Bodywork can help you maintain good health in several ways:

✔ It reduces tension and stress, both of which have strong links to pain.

Alleviating stress can help lessen (or possibly reduce altogether) the pain associated with various health conditions — and it's a well-known fact that stress and tension can present themselves in the form of physical conditions, such as headaches, muscle pain, and other problems.

✔ It stimulates the nervous system to release *endorphins,* those neurotransmitters that elevate a person's mood and create a sense of well-being.

✔ It eases the ups and downs of hormonal shifts, which are also impacted by changes in qi flow.

> ✔ It develops your awareness of the connection between your emotions and your physical self. With awareness, you can take control of the balance in your life.

Boosting self-awareness

Proper regular maintenance means that you must maintain a healthy, balanced qi, or energy, flow. Ideally, you maintain this balance at all times, or at least as much as possible. This means that you must be in tune with your systems as acutely as possible, so that you can immediately detect and address any slight disruptions or disturbances in your energy flow.

Your qi inevitably varies somewhat from day to day — it's just the natural cycle of ups and downs. Your qi is affected by a whole laundry list of factors: your emotional state, your surroundings, even the time of year (seasonal shifts). Any deviations in your regular routine (dietary changes, disruptions in your sleep pattern, and so on) can also affect the balance of your qi. For women, qi levels tend to fluctuate in relation to changing hormone levels throughout the month.

Bodywork routines nurture your senses, sharpening your ability to continuously assess the state of your energy. As you become more aware of your own body's natural balance, you're able to immediately recognize (and even anticipate) when something is "off" and take steps to restore harmony to your system before any serious complications appear. For example, if you know that your qi will be off-balance because you've been skimping on sleep lately, you may also know that you need to take certain steps — such as performing specific self-healing techniques — in order to restore the proper energy flow.

It's important that you acknowledge your ability to diagnose the state of your own qi. Too many people doubt their own instincts. You know your body better than anyone. Listen to the signals it gives you. If you have a hunch that something is off, you have a good chance of being right, even if you're not yet experiencing any obvious symptoms.

This self-awareness is really a gift. Rather than ignoring it, you should embrace it. This special insight into your own condition will help you spot the slightest imbalance and make necessary adjustments while the potential problem is still in its earliest stages.

Preventative Treatments to Reduce Future Concerns

Keeping your system in proper balance and harmony doesn't involve simply making adjustments after you notice changes in your qi. Equally important is taking the offensive and trying to *prevent* problems before they happen.

By encouraging your body's healthy energy flow and vitality on a regular basis, you can often prevent the stagnant state that causes many disruptions in qi and, inevitably, discomfort or pain.

Relieving stress, tension, and fatigue

Mental and emotional stress, along with physical tension and fatigue, can cause or contribute to a long list of painful problems and health concerns. By practicing the stress-reducing routines in this section, you can take a big step in heading off future problems. You can find the points you need in Figures 6-1, 6-2, and 6-3, and you can read about them in Table 6-1. If you're not sure how to measure *chon,* check out Chapter 3.

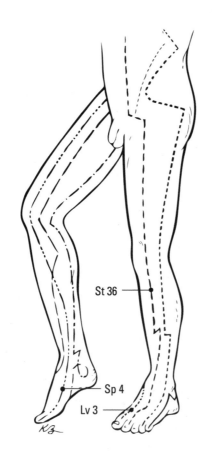

Figure 6-1:
Acupoints
on the legs
and feet.

St 36

Sp 4

Lv 3

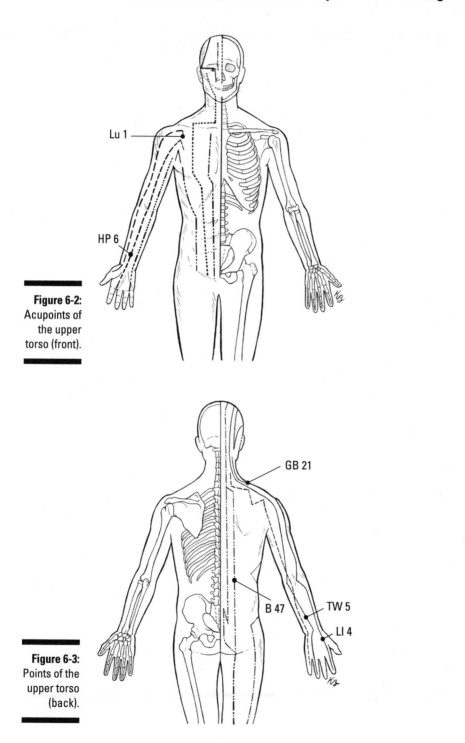

Figure 6-2:
Acupoints of
the upper
torso (front).

Figure 6-3:
Points of the
upper torso
(back).

Table 6-1		Points for Optimal Wellness	
Point Abbreviation	*Name of Point*	*How You Find It*	*Benefits*
St 36	Three Mile Point	Two chon down from the kneecap and four chon to the outside of the leg.	Strengthens and nourishes qi, relieves fatigue, and regulates energy flow.
Lv 3	Great Rushing	One chon from the base of the big toe, in the web-bing between the big and second toes.	This point is a powerful harmonizer that keeps qi flowing smoothly. Use it to invigorate and clear the system.
Sp 4	Grandfather-Grandson	This point is on the side of the inside of the foot, one chon behind the base of the big toe. Find the bone in the arch of the foot, hook your finger into the arch from underneath, and press upward.	This point supports and nourishes all aspects of the body-mind and balances circulation. Use for grounding and emotional balance while relieving worry and anxiety.
HP 6	Inner Gate	On the palm side of the arm, two chon above the wrist crease between the two tendons.	This point balances yin energy (see Chapter 1) and protects the heart meridian from excess stress. Use to release the chest and encourage deep breathing. Also good for nausea.
TW 5	Outer Gate	On the back side of the arm, two chon above the wrist crease between the two tendons.	Use to stimulate abundant energy flow and support immune function. Good for balancing yang energy.
LI 4*	Union Valley	In the webbing where the index finger and the thumb meet. If you close your finger and thumb, you'll find it at the bottom of the crease. You can pinch this point between your index finger and thumb.	Use to reduce muscle tension and relieve stress. Promotes downward flow of qi.

Point Abbreviation	Name of Point	How You Find It	Benefits
Lu 1	Central Treasury	This point is located on your rib cage, one chon down from where your arm meets your chest wall. Use your thumbs and press this point toward the breastbone.	Use to open the chest and promote deep breathing. Increases blood and qi flow, and balances emotion.
B 47	Will's Chamber	Place your hands on your waist with your fingers pointing forward and your thumbs pointing backward. Slide your thumbs toward your spine. When you hit the erector muscles, you'll find a sore spot. It's about three chon away from the spine.	Use to distribute qi to all the meridians. Supports the whole body, and relieves back tension.
GB 21	Shoulder Well	In the top of the shoulder, halfway between the point of your shoulder and the base of your neck. In the belly of the muscle.	Use to relieve stress and tension. Encourages downward-flowing qi.

* Never use this point during pregnancy.

The routine in this section — which requires all of 20 minutes — will help keep you healthy if you do it on a regular basis. It focuses on stimulating and regulating qi flow and establishes harmony throughout your body. You can hold all these points on a friend, too. First lead the receiver through the stretching and breathing exercises that follow:

1. **Sit quietly in a chair or in a cross-legged position on the floor. Take three deep, balancing breaths from your belly to help energize your body. At the same time, try to ground and center yourself.**

   Refer to Chapter 2 for an explanation of these important techniques.

2. **Continue the belly breathing while stretching your whole body:**

    • Stand up and take your arms up over your head while breathing in and stretch backward as far as it's comfortable (don't overstretch and hurt yourself!). Hold for the count of three.

    • Exhale as you bend forward, stretching your arms to the floor. Be a rag doll and hold this stretch for the count of three.

    • Inhale as you stand back up; bring your arms over your head and lean to the side, exhaling while you lean. Hold for a count of three. Breathe in as you straighten up, and repeat on the other side.

    • Repeat the whole sequence three times to fully open all meridian channels.

After you warm up, you're ready to begin the pressure-point routine. Ask the receiver to lie down face-up on a comfortable mat or table before you begin addressing the acupoints. Before you begin, identify the points in Figures 6-1, 6-2, and 6-3. If you're working on yourself, you can do all these while sitting in a chair. Throughout the session, you may need to ask the receiver to move once or twice. You use a bilateral approach on the legs and back points and a one-meridian-at-a-time approach on the arms, just because it's hard to hold points bilaterally on the arms.

Press the following sequences of points using alternating pressure for full points and sustained pressure for empty points:

1. **Use the bilateral approach on points St 36, Lv 3, and Sp 4.**

   Hold each point on both sides at the same time for 2 to 3 minutes. Repeat the sequence two to three times until all points feel equal.

2. **Use the one-meridian-at-a-time approach on the points HP 6, TW 5, and LI 4.**

   Starting with either arm, press each point one at a time, pulsing the pressure on each for about 30 seconds, and then moving on. Repeat the sequence three times on each arm.

3. **Use the bilateral approach on the points Lu 1, B 47, and GB 21.**

   Hold each point for 2 to 3 minutes. Repeat the sequence three times.

4. **Finish the treatment by lying quietly and relaxing (or by having the receiver lie quietly and relax).**

   You may notice warmth and tingling throughout your body and an overall sense of openness and well-being. Focus your thoughts on attracting health, harmony, and happiness.

You can follow this routine with the reflexology routine for well-being, which we explain in the next section, or simply spend time relaxing.

Reflexology routine for total wellness

Total wellness means just that — wellness in all your parts: physical, mental, and spiritual. The following routine stimulates all parts of the foot and therefore all parts of the body-mind; if you want to focus more on particular areas, use the reflex map in Figure 6-4 as your guide.

Follow these steps for a comprehensive session:

1. **Start by washing and drying your feet.**

   You can turn this step into a ritual by adding creams or oils and pampering yourself.

   You can perform this routine on a friend with simple adaptations. Sit down with the receiver in a chair that's opposite yours. Hold your friend's foot in your lap. Be sure he's warm and comfortable. Or, have him lie face-up on a mat with a large pillow under his knees. Lift each foot one at a time. Proceed in the same way you did for yourself, paying attention to the receiver's feedback. Of course, all you may hear is *ahh* and *ohhh,* but you can consider those affirmations of approval.

2. **If you haven't already stretched and performed deep breathing exercises, do some deep belly breathing now. See Chapter 2 for more about deep breathing routines.**

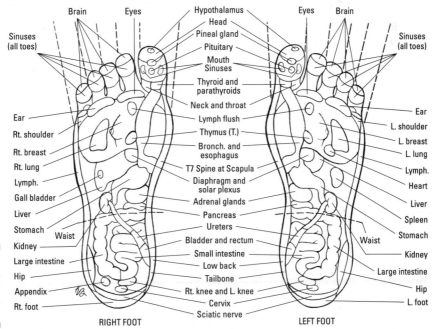

Figure 6-4:
Reflexology map for total wellness.

3. **Sit in a chair or on a bed and cross your leg so that you can hold your foot in your lap. Use the foot rolling technique (see Chapter 4) to loosen up any qi-flow restrictions.**

4. **Use the foot stripping technique (see Chapter 4).**

   Repeat in rows until you reach your heel. Do this three or four times.

5. **Use the circular motion technique all over your foot.**

   If you have a tender place, look it up on your foot map. Give these areas extra attention with stretching and circular pressure. Hold these points with sustained pressure, and then follow sustained pressure with pulsing pressure. Continue on each point for several minutes or until it's no longer sore.

6. **Repeat all steps on the other foot.**

7. **End with 5 to 10 minutes of relaxation, breathing deeply and noticing the relaxation and well-being spreading through your body.**

   Relaxation is the time when your body integrates the flow of qi.

Chapter 7

Balancing Emotions for Well-Being

*E*motions have a huge impact on how you feel, how much enthusiasm and appetite you have for life, and how healthy you are in general. This chapter explores the way emotions, thoughts, attitudes, and beliefs impact your qi and affect your health and well-being. You also discover how to shift the unconscious patterns that get in your way and cause your body discomfort, by using simple but powerful tools on yourself or on friends and family. Just remember, everything changes in its own time — you can't force the emotional well-being, but you sure can encourage it!

Emotions Happen in the Body

You were probably taught that emotions happen in the brain as a chemical process, right? You may be surprised to learn that an increasing segment of the scientific community is now embracing the belief that emotions are *somatic,* or body events. Instead of happening in the brain, they happen in the body. This may be a new way of thinking, but it makes sense.

Imagine the last time you felt really sad. Let yourself deeply feel the sadness as you remember the event surrounding it. Where do you feel sadness? Most people feel it in their heart, or chest area. Another emotion people feel in the chest area is love. Think about a person or animal who you really love; imagine the last time you enjoyed this person or animal. Really immerse yourself in the memory and let the feeling of love grow and grow. Where do you feel it? Exactly! On the other hand, when was the last time you felt anxious? Did you get butterflies in your stomach? Anxiety is usually felt in the stomach, or solar plexus. Most people feel emotions somewhere in the torso, and, although everyone is different, many people share the same association between what they feel and where they feel it.

Generally, most people trust their feelings and perceptions. If you feel pain coming from your left toe, you look at your left toe to see what's wrong. You don't imagine that the pain is really in your head and that you're accidentally feeling it in your toe, do you? But that's what people do with emotions. Even though you feel the emotion in your body, you think it's coming from your head! Actually the chemicals in the brain that are associated with emotions are found in all parts of the body and can be made by any cell.

Some scientists, like Dr. Candace Pert, now think that one of the functions of emotion is to communicate between the body and the mind. Research conducted over the last decade shows that chemicals of emotion are made by cells throughout the body, and these chemicals travel to the brain, giving the brain information about the body. The process works in both directions because brain cells also create emotion-related chemicals that travel to the body. This is the basis of mind-body medicine.

If you find this concept as fascinating as we do, check out these books: *Molecules of Emotion: The Science Behind Mind-Body Medicine* by Candace B. Pert (Simon & Schuster) and *Bodymind* by Ken Dychtwald (Tarcher Putman).

Feelings and their locations

Although everyone is different, many people share the same association between what they feel and where they feel it. You may notice an association in the metaphors people use. For example, when you feel grief, your heart is broken; when you're anxious, you get butterflies in your stomach; and when something makes you angry, it's galling. I'm sure you can think of several more examples. Here are some common associations between areas in the torso and emotions — both balanced and unbalanced:

Location	Balanced emotion	Unbalanced emotion
Pelvic bowel	Safety	Mortal fear/terror
Lower abdomen	Pride	Shame/guilt
Upper abdomen	Personal power	Anxiety/anger
Chest	Love/happiness	Grief/sadness

Smile at your organs

A Taoist saying goes like this: "Smiling causes the organs to secrete sweet substances; frowning causes the organs to secrete sour substances." Many people take this saying to heart and start each day by taking five minutes to smile at every organ in their body. Try it! You may be surprised.

Eastern medicine is way ahead of the game! The idea that mind and emotions are important in illness is integral to traditional Chinese medicine and dates back more than 2,000 years. In this medicine, emotions are considered to be generated in the body and transmitted on qi. Imbalances or emotional stress can cause muscle tension and problems with organ function. Acupressure is an ideal tool for balancing emotions and thus promoting wellness.

Emotions and Meridians

Each meridian governs an organ and is generally named after the organ it governs. Each organ generates, stores, or distributes an emotional quality. Yin organs and meridians generate emotions, and their yang partners distribute the emotional information to the rest of the body-mind. Meridians and organs generate both balanced and unbalanced emotions; however, people typically focus on the unbalanced aspects. Naturally, if things are going well, you leave them alone. The only reason you balance a meridian is if it's out of balance. Before we go too much further, take a look at the following associations:

- ✔ **Liver:** Generates anger, frustration, irritability, and resentment; deals with planning and decision-making

- ✔ **Gall Bladder:** Expresses anger and depression (anger against self); deals with executing the plans and decisions of the liver

- ✔ **Lung:** Generates grief; deals with boundaries (what to take in, what to let go of)

- ✔ **Large Intestine:** Expresses grief; maintains the boundaries

- ✔ **Kidney:** Generates fear; stores ancestral energy or genetic material

- ✔ **Bladder:** Expresses fear in fight or flight behavior; manages genetic information

- ✔ **Spleen:** Generates worry and pensiveness; deals with memory and reminiscence

- ✔ **Stomach:** Expresses worry; affects memory; pursues or neglects self-care

- ✔ **Heart:** Generates joy; imbalance is overjoy (overstimulation), anxiety, and shock; deals with knowing your path, passion, and spiritual center

- ✔ **Small Intestine:** Distributes emotions of the heart; assimilates information

- ✔ **Heart Protector:** Protects the heart from excess and shock. The heart protector is an extra meridian that doesn't have an organ association per se but relates to the *pericardium,* a fluid-filled membrane that surrounds the heart, protecting it from injury and infection. It's considered a second heart meridian.

- ✔ **Triple Warmer:** Distributes emotions of the heart and information of the small intestine through the "three heaters," or burners, of the torso. The TW doesn't have an actual organ association, but is associated with the three energy centers and nerve complexes of the torso — the brachial plexus, solar plexus, and sacral plexus.

You may want to look at Chapter 3 to refresh your memory on the meridians.

When you consider emotional balance, look at what's generating the emotion and how it's being expressed. You can use this information to determine your healing routine. For example, if you're worried and anxious, be sure to check the balance of the stomach and spleen meridians when creating your healing plan. The reverse works, too — for example, if you have a stomachache, you may wonder what you're worried about. Connecting the stomachache to an emotion can help eliminate the tension you're holding especially if you're using acupressure or reflexology to balance the meridian or organ that governs the emotion at the same time. So the next time you're feeling a physical pain, see whether you can find an emotional association while balancing the appropriate points. You can find the points you need in the session plans in Chapters 6 through 18.

How Your Thinking Affects Your Qi

Every thought you think produces a reaction in the body. If you hear a noise in the basement and think it's an intruder, your body generates fear. Fear is distributed through the body with a chemical cascade that sends a message to every cell to get ready for action. But wait — suddenly you remember that you left the window open and what you hear is the wind. Whew, harmless! As your thinking changes, your emotion changes to relief and, slowly, your pounding heart slows down. This is just one example of how your thoughts affect your body by generating emotions.

The more aware you are of how your thoughts and emotions create body reactions, the more control you have over your wellness. Negative thoughts generate emotions that restrict qi flow, raise blood pressure, create digestive upset, and undermine the immune system. Positive thoughts open the flood gates and allow qi to flow freely and evenly through the body. This promotes healthy function of all organs.

Eastern medicine believes that thought directs your qi. We talk about attention in Chapter 2. Where you put your attention is where your qi goes. If you always put your attention on what isn't working, your energy supports what isn't working. Here's an example: Co-author Synthia has a client with high blood pressure. She worries about how high it is and takes her blood pressure several times every day. When it's high, she's anxious because it's high. When it's low, she's anxious that it will rise. This type of worry raises her blood pressure. This is an example of sending your qi with your mind to produce unhealthy effects. A better approach would be, to send positive thoughts about how well your body works. This directs the qi to support healthy function.

The Transformational Power of Acupressure and Reflexology

Acupressure and reflexology have the power to transform your life. Fears and insecurities that hold you back can be transformed into strengths. Attitudes and beliefs that undermine your confidence can be shifted into positive outlooks. If you take the time to explore your attitudes, emotions, and thoughts while using acupressure points, your emotions will clear, your qi will shift, and your thinking will become more positive.

Suppose you have an energy block in the gall bladder meridian in your left leg. Maybe you're having trouble making a certain decision, and this has built up in your meridian. Every time you think of how much your leg bothers you, you send energy to the block. This energy isn't necessarily a good thing. Sending more energy can add to the block, building greater pressure. On the other hand, sending your attention to the blocked area and exploring it can produce the opposite effect. It can release the block and allow stagnant qi to move. How does this happen? Actually, a lot of blocks occur because you have unconscious beliefs or unresolved emotions, and exploring them helps to resolve them.

You can find many great books on the subject of changing your attitudes and emotions with positive thinking. Reading these books while using acupressure for emotional well-being has tremendous power to transform your life. The best book for using acupressure to transform emotions is *Acupressure Way of Health: Jin Shin Do* by Iona Marsaa Teeguarden (Japan Publications).

Reflexology can also help shift emotions and release qi. When you use reflexology and acupressure together, the two join forces and increase the effectiveness of both. Reflexology doesn't have a list of associated emotions, but you can borrow the associations from acupressure and apply them to reflexology. A British study in the 1990s showed that reflexology provided beneficial emotional effects. The study, titled "Reflexology meets Emotional Needs," was reported in the *International Journal of Alternative and Complementary Medicine* in November 1996. According to the study, reflexology provided improvements both physically and emotionally, including improved self-esteem, motivation, and self-confidence.

Using the tools of acupressure and reflexology allows you to let go of the experiences you've stored that limit the way you express your true self. It's a pathway to being more fully who you are and who you want to be. So what are you waiting for? Read the following sections and get to work!

Balancing Points for Emotional Well-Being

Emotional well-being is a whole body event and incorporates all the meridians. Remember that the meridians are all different bends in the same river, so an imbalance in one essentially creates an imbalance through the entire system. Like optimal wellness, emotional well-being is more than an absence of symptoms like depression or frustration. It's an appetite for life. It includes feelings of confidence and self-worth, a desire to fulfill one's dreams, and the motivation to do so.

Working major points on all the meridians would take way too long, but fortunately, the meridians have special points that have a balancing effect over the entire meridian. They're sort of like primer points, priming the entire pathway. They're called *source points* and they balance a meridian whether it's empty or full so that it can be used any time. All the source points are located on the hands and feet, making it easy to give a good self-balancing session. You can optimize your results by practicing positive thinking and affirmations while holding and pressing points.

Be sure to get everything ready first. You need your bone-locating and point-locating charts from Chapter 3. And don't forget to have fun!

A good reference book for positive thinking and mind-body associations is *You Can Heal Your Life* by Louise L. Hay (Full Circle Publishing, Ltd.). To find more of the many great books and Web sites out there, search the Web with keywords such as *positive thinking*, *affirmations*, and *right thinking*.

Acupressure routine

Familiarize yourself with the following points, which you use in the acupressure routine for emotional well-being. You can find all the points for the routine in Figures 7-1, 7-2, and 7-3, and you can read about them in Table 7-1. Chapter 3 tells you how to measure *chon*.

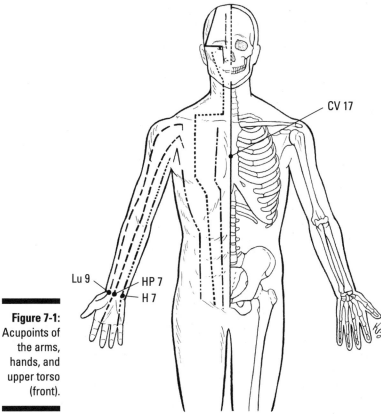

Figure 7-1: Acupoints of the arms, hands, and upper torso (front).

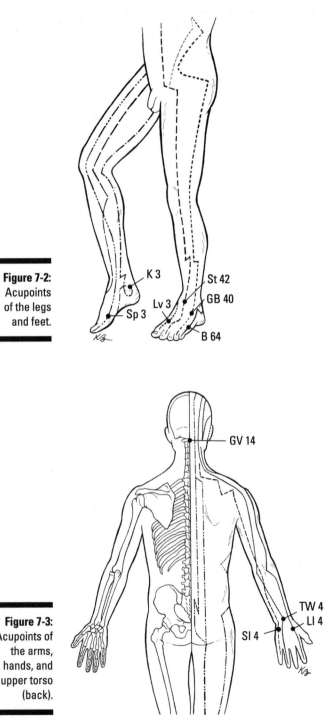

Figure 7-2:
Acupoints
of the legs
and feet.

Figure 7-3:
Acupoints of
the arms,
hands, and
upper torso
(back).

Table 7-1		A Guide to Source Points	
Point Abbreviation	**Name of Point**	**How You Find It**	**Benefits**
Lu 9	Great Abyss	On the palm surface of the hand, halfway between the outside of the wrist and the first joint of the thumb in the wrist crease.	Source point for the lung. Regulates and tonifies lung qi and yin qi.
LI 4*	Union Valley	In the webbing where the index finger and the thumb meet. If you close your finger and thumb, you'll find it at the bottom of the crease. You can pinch this point between your index finger and thumb.	Source point for the large intestine. Regulates large intestine qi and moistens the colon. Stimulates downward-flowing energy.
Sp 3	Supreme Whiteness	Go to the side of the inside of the foot. Find the base of the big toe. Slide into the depression between the base of the big toe and the metatarsal bone, staying on the side of the foot.	Source point for the spleen. Regulates and tonifies the spleen, and clears heat.
St 42	Surging Yang	Go to the backside of the foot to the second and third toes. Trace between the metatarsal bones up to where they meet. Keep going to the highest point on the top of the foot.	Source point for the stomach. Regulates the stomach and calms the spirit.
H 7	Spirit Gate	Palm side up, go to the outer edge of the wrist, at the crease between the ulna bones and the carpal bones.	Source point for the heart. Regulates and tonifies the heart. Calms the spirit and balances emotions.

(continued)

Table 7-1 *(continued)*

Point Abbreviation	Name of Point	How You Find It	Benefits
SI 4	Wrist Bone	Go to the little finger side of the hand at the wrist between the two bones and slightly toward the fingers. Your pressure will be on the side ridge.	Source point for the small intestine. Invigorates qi.
K 3	Great Ravine	Go to the highest point of the inner anklebone and slide backward halfway to the Achilles tendon.	Source point for the kidney. Tonifies, regulates, and stabilizes kidney qi.
B 64	Capitol Bone	Go to the outer side of the foot, find the base of the small toe, and slide toward the ankle one chon to the top of the metatarsal bone.	Source point for the bladder. Regulates the bladder and calms the spirit.
HP 7	Great Mound	Go to the palm side of the wrist crease and find the point halfway between the inside and outside of the wrist between the two tendons.	Source point for the heart protector. Regulates and clears excess fire from the heart. Calms and sedates the body-mind.
TW 4	Yang Pool	Go to the back of the hand to the wrist and find the point in the middle of the crease halfway between the inside and outside of the wrist.	Source point for the triple warmer. Dispels wind and heat.
GB 40	Hill Ruins	Go to the outer anklebone, drop one chon below the anklebone and one chon in front of the anklebone to find a little depression.	Source point for the gall bladder. Regulates and transforms gall bladder qi.

Point Abbreviation	Name of Point	How You Find It	Benefits
Lv 3	Great Rushing	On the top side of the foot, go between the big and second toes; trace up the webbing between the metatarsal bones until the bones come together, forming a depression.	Source point for the liver. Regulates and tonifies liver qi. Provides an overall calming effect.
CV 17	Upper Sea of Qi	Go to the exact center of the breastbone, almost halfway between top and bottom, slightly closer to the bottom.	Meeting point for the conception vessel. Calms the spirit and harmonizes yin qi.
GV 14	Great Hammer	Between the last vertebra in the neck and the first vertebra in the back.	Meeting point for the governing vessel. Facilitates and invigorates qi flow and harmonizes yang qi.

* Never use this point during pregnancy.

Focus on the points in Table 7-1 when you're performing this routine that encourages emotional well-being.

1. **Start every session with grounding, centering, and belly breathing (see Chapter 2 for details).**

2. **Stretch your whole body while continuing the belly breathing.**

   Even though all the source points are on the hands and feet, they affect the whole body, making it a whole-body treatment, so go ahead and use the following stretches to start out:

   • Take your arms up over your head while breathing in and stretch backward as far as you comfortably can (don't overstretch and hurt yourself!). Hold for the count of three.

   • Exhale as you bend forward, stretching your arms to the floor. Be a rag doll and hold this stretch for the count of three.

   • Inhale as you stand back up; bring your arms over your head and lean to the side, exhaling while you lean. Hold.

   • Breathe in as you straighten up and repeat to the other side.

   • Repeat the whole sequence three times to fully open all meridian channels.

3. **Balance the meridians on both sides of the body.**

   - To balance the points, press each one with a deep, sustained pressure for three minutes or until you feel a change. Then pulse pressure on the point for another one to two minutes. (See Chapter 4 for more info.)

   - If a 24-point session is too long, find each point but treat only the ones that feel sore.

4. **End your session by pressing CV 17 and GV 14 on the Central Channel.**

   The front point on the breastbone connects with all yin meridians in the body. The point on the back of the neck connects all yang meridians in the body. Ending your session with these yin/yang balancing points puts the icing on a great, overall, emotionally balancing routine.

   - Press CV 17 at the same time as GV 14. These two points promote great relaxation.

   - Hold the two points with medium to light sustained pressure for three to four minutes.

5. **Relax quietly for five to ten minutes, paying attention to any insight you may have about your stress.**

Reflexology routine

Emotional well-being is a whole-body event physically, mentally, and spiritually. The following routine adds to the routine for total wellness in Chapter 6, stimulating all parts of the foot and therefore all parts of the body-mind. See Chapter 4 for explanations on how to perform the various techniques.

1. **Start by washing and drying your feet.**

2. **If you haven't already stretched and performed deep breathing exercises, do some grounding, centering, and deep belly breathing now. (See Chapter 2 for details.)**

3. **Sit in a chair or on a bed and cross your leg so that you can hold your foot in your lap.**

4. **Roll your foot back and forth in your hand, loosening up any restriction.**

5. **Perform foot stripping all over your foot.**

   Start this step at the top of the foot and repeat in rows until you reach your heel. Do this three or four times.

6. **Start at your big toe, and use your thumbs to press and release while thumb-walking down a row from your toe to your heel (see Chapter 4).**

Make a row for each toe. This stimulates all the reflex zones.

7. **Add circular motions.**

You can use two approaches to this step, and both are great:

- You can simply use the circular pressure over certain reflex points on the feet (see Figure 7-4), taking note of which ones are tender, crystallized, hard, empty, and so on. Work on those points, adding and releasing pressure until they change. As that happens, your emotional tension will change, too.

- Or, consider what emotional state you're in. If you're angry, use circular motions and pulsating pressure over the liver and gall bladder areas of your feet. You can do this for any emotion, using the acupressure organ associations.

8. **Repeat with the other foot.**

Don't forget that you can perform this routine on a friend with simple adaptations. Check out Chapter 6 for details, and be sure to pay attention to your friend's feedback.

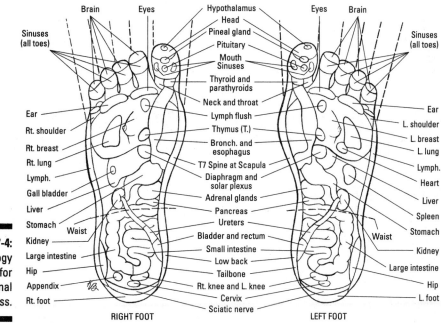

Figure 7-4: Reflexology map for emotional wellness.

Chapter 8

Treating Emotional Upset

*E*ver wonder why people spend so much time trying to control their emotions? What if, instead of trying to get rid of them, you tried to understand their message? In this chapter, we tell you why emotions have so much influence over how you feel physically. We show you ways to keep anxiety, stress, and other emotional issues from having a negative impact on your health. Finally, we give you insight on techniques that can help you alleviate pain and other physical symptoms that may have been triggered by emotional factors. Although we don't cover the fundamental acupressure techniques in this chapter, you can find all the basics in Chapter 4.

Stress: The Good, the Bad, and the Consuming

The majority of physical and emotional tension you experience comes from stress. Chronic stress contributes to many debilitating health problems, such as heart disease, high cholesterol, chronic fatigue, musculoskeletal problems, emotional distress, and terminal illness.

As bad as stress can be for health, it's also an essential ingredient for growth and expansion. Without physical stress, you can't develop strong muscles and bones or cardiovascular fitness. Without psychological stress, you may not be challenged to develop your abilities and discover your highest potential.

So when does good stress become bad stress? Stress becomes harmful when you don't allow yourself recovery time; when tense muscles aren't allowed to rest; when you rush from one demand to another; when you don't have control over the forces in your life. Growth-oriented stress has periods of demand and periods of rest. Muscles can't lift weights all day long; they need time to rest and repair damage; time to restore nutrient and oxygen levels. Without rest, your muscles get weak and become a site for potential injury. Psychologically, the information you take in can integrate during your rest time, resulting in a new insight or potential skill. If you're always pushing, you don't have enough time to learn from what you're doing. Harmful stress is a signal that you're out of balance and out of touch with yourself.

Telling the difference between good stress and bad stress can be a major challenge. Ask yourself whether the things you do give you energy or take it away. How would your life be different if you had fewer demands? Everyone is different; you may be the type of person who thrives on deadlines and high-pressure situations. No one but you knows whether the level of stress in your life is good for you.

From the perspective of Chinese medicine, stress can be disruptive to the harmonious flow of qi, unbalancing the meridians. One easy way to reduce the impact of stress on your health is to take acupressure breaks and restore your smooth flow of qi. It's a great way to relax and rejuvenate even if you have only a few short minutes to practice. In the end, to be in touch with yourself requires time to connect inwardly. Pressure point therapies are an ideal way to do this.

Stress-free pressure points in the head, neck, and shoulders

If you're like the majority of the population, stress tends to build up in the muscles of your shoulders and neck, causing neck pain and headaches. Table 8-1 provides pressure points that are great for reducing mental and emotional stress and relieving the physical effects of excess tension (if you're not sure how to measure *chon,* go to Chapter 3). Find the points in Figures 8-1, 8-2, and 8-3.

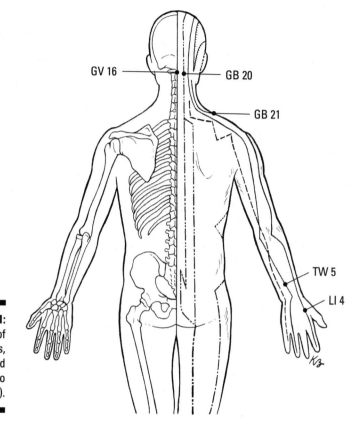

Figure 8-1:
Acupoints of
the arms,
hands, and
upper torso
(back).

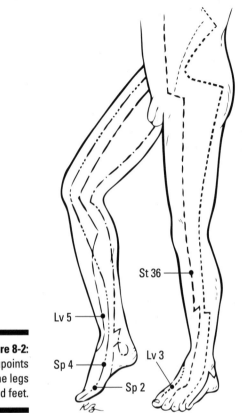

St 36

Lv 5

Figure 8-2:
Acupoints
of the legs
and feet.

Sp 4

Lv 3

Sp 2

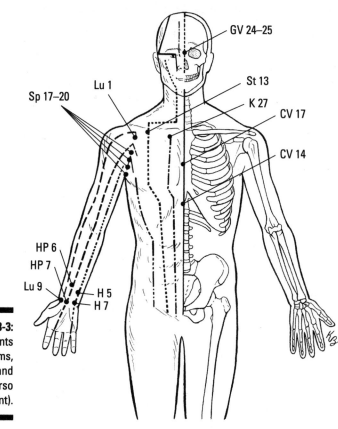

Figure 8-3:
Acupoints
of the arms,
head, and
upper torso
(front).

Table 8-1		Stress-Relieving Points for Head, Neck, and Shoulders	
Point Abbreviation	*Name of Point*	*How You Find It*	*Benefits*
GB 20	Wind Pool	Along the ridge of your occipital bone on the back of your head, halfway between your ear and spine; between the two muscles that come together.	Subdues liver meridian; used for tension headaches and migraines.
GB 21	Shoulder Well	In the top of the shoulder, halfway between the point of your shoulder and the base of your neck. In the belly of the muscle.	Use to reduce stiffness and pain of the neck, shoulder, and upper back.
LI 4*	Union Valley	In the webbing between your thumb and index finger. It's traditionally located at the crease where your thumb and finger meet when you hold your fingers straight out and close your fingers and thumb together.	Reduces muscular tension, and harmonizes the flow of qi.
Lv 3	Great Rushing	On the top side of the foot, go between the big and second toes; trace up the webbing between the metatarsal bones until the bones come together, forming a depression.	Rebalances the liver meridian, which assists the smooth flow of qi throughout the body. Provides an overall calming effect.

Point Abbreviation	Name of Point	How You Find It	Benefits
HP 7	Great Mound	Palm side of the wrist in the middle of the wrist crease between the two tendons.	Protects the heart and spirit from the emotional impact of excess stress. Clears excess fire from the heart. Calms and sedates the body-mind.
H 7	Spirit Gate	On the palm side of the wrist, in the wrist crease, directly under the little finger.	Calms the mind and emotions.
GV 24–25	Yintang (an extra point on the govern- ing vessel meridian)	On the bridge of the nose, between the eyebrows.	Calms the mind and emotions, and sedates qi.

*Never use this point during pregnancy.

You can simply hold the points or use the following routine:

1. **Belly breathe while centering and grounding (refer to Chapter 2).**

2. **Wrap a towel around your neck for some support, and then stretch by rolling your head in a full circle, three times in both directions. Stop anywhere it feels sore and hold the stretch for 20 seconds.**

3. **Using bilateral holds, press both GB 20s and then both GB 21s. Use sustained pressure if the point feels empty, or alternating pressure if the point feels full.**

4. **Alternately hold LI 4 on each hand. Use sustained pressure, or alternating pressure as indicated.**

5. **Use bilateral holds for both Lv 3s.**

6. **Alternately hold HP 7 and H 7 on each hand.**

7. **End by holding GV 24–25 between the eyebrows with gently sustained pressure for one to three minutes.**

8. **Spend a few minutes relaxing quietly and paying attention to any insight you may have about your stress.**

Face points for letting go

People often say things like, "I know something's wrong; I can see it written all over your face." Of course you know that you hold stress in your face; you can see the effects when you look in the mirror. This look is the effect of long-term, unrelenting stress! Table 8-2 shows you points to relieve face tension. Refer to Figure 8-1 and check out Figure 8-4 to locate the points.

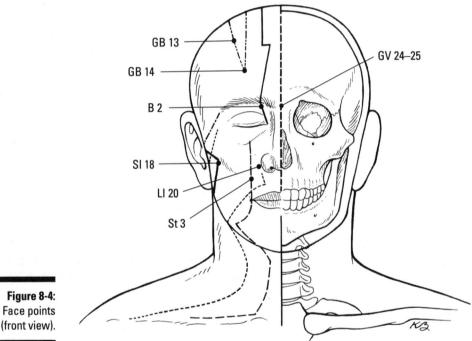

Figure 8-4:
Face points
(front view).

Table 8-2		Stress-Relieving Points for the Face	
Point Abbreviation	*Name of Point*	*How You Find It*	*Benefits*
GB 14	Yang White	Go to the middle of your eyebrow, and then go one chon above your eyebrow in your forehead.	Relieves frontal headaches and eye strain.
B 2	Bright Light	At the inner corner of your eyebrow, pressing into the orbit bone.	Relieves frontal headaches, face tension, and eye strain.
LI 20	Welcome Fragrance	Just outside the nostril, pressing up into the cheekbone.	Alleviates sinus headaches.
St 3	Great Bone Hole	Slide your finger from the outside of the nostril along the cheekbone to the lowest point of the bone. Press up into the bone from underneath.	Relieves face pain and swelling and sinusitis.
SI 18	Cheekbone Hole	Draw a line horizontally from the bottom of your nose to the depression in front of your ear. Then drop a line from the outside corner of your eye. SI 18 is located in the depression at the crossing of these lines.	Relieves face pain and facial nerve pain as well as swelling.
GB 20	Wind Pool	Along the ridge of your occipital bone halfway between your ear and spine; between the two muscles that come together.	Alleviates tension headaches and migraines.

(continued)

Table 8-2 *(continued)*

Point Abbreviation	Name of Point	How You Find It	Benefits
GV 16	Wind Mansion	Located in the depression in the center of your occipital bone where your spine enters your skull. It's very tender, so be gentle. To release tension here, place both of your index fingers in the depression, apply pressure and gently pull your fingers away from each other, stretching the strong tendons that cross the skull at this point.	Alleviates stiff neck and headache.
LI 4*	Union Valley	This point is in the webbing between your thumb and index finger. It's traditionally located at the crease where your thumb and finger meet when you hold your fingers straight out and close your fingers and thumb together.	Regulates qi flow. Used for tension headaches, migraines, and neuralgia.

* Never use this point during pregnancy.

You can use these points anytime, anywhere, or you can make a special time to use this de-stressing face routine. To maximize effectiveness, find all the points before you begin so that you don't stress out trying to find them during the session. Before you address the points, though, we recommend a soothing relaxation treatment as a warm-up:

1. **Put a washcloth in a pan of hot (not boiling!) water and put it next to the area where you'll be working.**

   Add a chamomile tea bag for an added relaxation treat.

2. **Contract all the muscles in your face; scrunch up your mouth, your eyes, and your forehead.**

   Squeeze all the muscles as tight as you can.

3. **Open your mouth, stretch your lips, and widen your eyes.**

   Open everything as far as you can.

4. **Relax and place your hands over the sides of your face, covering as much of your face as you can. Pull your skin upward, and then downward; forward and then backward.**

   Hold each stretched position for 30 seconds to one minute.

5. **Wring out the washcloth, lie down or lean back in your chair, and place the washcloth over your face.**

6. **Take a few minutes to relax all the muscles in your body.**

   Give yourself an opportunity to enjoy breathing in and breathing out; listen to the sounds around you; let yourself be present without having to do anything.

   You can rewarm the washcloth in the pan of hot water as many times as you want to.

7. **When you finish the warm washcloth treatment, use the bilateral approach and hold each point from Table 8-2 on both sides of your face at the same time.**

   Start in order, beginning with GB 14 on the forehead. Hold each point with sustained or alternating pressure for 30 seconds to 3 minutes.

Reflexology to the stress rescue

Reflexology can be a lifesaver in alleviating the uncomfortable physical effects that stress and anxiety often cause. We recommend using this routine as a way to combat the toll that stress takes on your body. Note also that using reflexology has the added benefit of relieving one of the most stressed parts of your body — your feet. Choosing between reflexology and acupressure isn't hard — they both work great, so do whichever feels best to you! See Chapter 4 for details on how to perform the various techniques.

1. **Wash and dry your feet.**

2. **If you haven't already stretched and performed deep breathing exercises, do some deep belly breathing now.**

3. **Sit in a chair or on a bed and cross your leg so that you can hold your foot in your lap.**

4. **Roll your foot back and forth in your hand, loosening up any restriction.**

5. **Use foot stripping to further open the reflex zones.**

6. **Thumb-walk and massage the entire foot, paying special attention to any soreness that you find.**

7. **Ask yourself how stress affects you as you work the spine, shoulder, and neck reflex points, and again as you work the stomach reflex points (see Figure 8-5).**

   Do you get tense shoulders or a backache as you work your spine, shoulder, and neck? Do you get butterflies in your stomach as you work on that area?

   You can use circular motions on all the reflex areas for your own stress patterns.

8. **End with thumb-walking and circular motions to the solar plexus and the adrenals, which are both important forces in managing stress.**

9. **Repeat with the other foot.**

10. **Relax and fully experience the sensations of reduced stress, such as decreased muscle tension, less mental chatter, and greater well-being.**

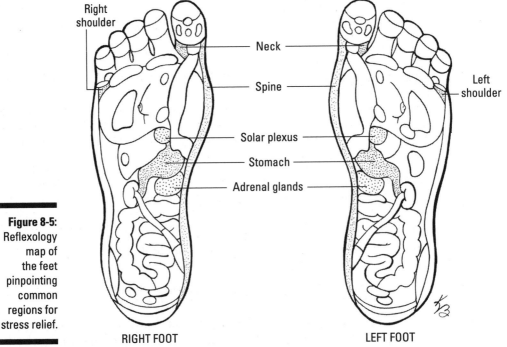

Figure 8-5:
Reflexology map of the feet pinpointing common regions for stress relief.

RIGHT FOOT   LEFT FOOT

Getting Hold of Worry and Anxiety

Mental concentration consumes more energy than any other function in the body. In Chinese medicine, excessive thinking, or worry, deprives the rest of the body of vital qi. On the other hand, worry is a natural part of living. Like stress, worry has a productive side. Worry may prompt you to prepare for an upcoming challenge. It can alert you to areas where you may not be performing up to standard. It can keep you attentive to situations that may be dangerous, allowing you to avoid harm.

Worry becomes nonproductive when it's consuming and no longer results in positive action. Unfortunately, a lot of worry is nothing more than your brain rehashing the same information over and over again, without creating any change. Worry of this kind drains you of energy and steals energy from the rest of the meridians and organs.

The stomach and spleen meridians govern mental activity and worry (see Chapter 3 for more info). Balanced qi in these meridians allows for sharp intellect, attention to important details, and the proper "digestion" and analysis of information. When these meridians are unbalanced, you may have a hard time analyzing information, which is the root of much worry.

Anxiety is related to worry but is less mentally focused. Anxiety can result from feeling out of control, or at the mercy of events around you. While worry is usually focused on the future, anxiety is more immediate. If you've ever had an anxiety attack, you know how uncomfortable it can be. You may experience a pounding heart with shortness of breath and extreme emotional agitation.

In meridian theory, anxiety is an imbalance in qi flow in the heart meridian. In Chapter 3 we talk about the meridians being one continuous river of qi that changes names when it changes directions. Well, interestingly, the spleen section of the river turns into the heart section of the river. Anxiety is sometimes a reflection of excessive worry holding energy in the spleen and causing a deficiency in the heart channel.

Moderate fluctuations in emotions are normal, but you should take any major roller-coaster swings in emotions seriously and mention them to your doctor. Major emotional fluctuations could indicate a medical disorder that requires treatment (possibly including medication, therapy, or a combination of the two).

Acupoints for mental relaxation

Become familiar with the points in Table 8-3, which you use in the routine that follows. Refer to Figures 8-1, 8-2, 8-3, and 8-4 to locate the points.

Table 8-3		Acupoints to Relieve Worry	
Point Abbreviation	*Name of Point*	*How You Find It*	*Benefits*
GB 13	Mind Root	Go to the outer edge of the eyebrow, and then move up one palm-width to a point just inside the hairline.	Calms the mind, and relieves anxiety.
GB 21	Shoulder Well	In the top of the shoulder, halfway between the point of your shoulder and the base of your neck. In the belly of the muscle.	Used for stiffness and pain in the neck, shoulder, and upper back. Relieves frustration, irritability, and fatigue.
St 13	Qi Door	Just underneath the collarbone, halfway between the breast-bone and the point of the shoulder.	Opens the chest, increasing oxygen and qi flow to the upper body and head. Can help mental focus, clarity, and relaxation.
Sp 17 Sp 18 Sp 19 Sp 20	Food Hole Celestial Ravine Chest Village All-Around Flourishing	These four points are between the ribs on the side of the rib cage, starting at rib four, at the bottom of the armpit.	Regulates chest qi, and harmonizes extremes.
K 27	Shu Mansion	Under the collarbone in the depression next to the breastbone.	Used for headaches due to mental strain, mental fatigue, dis-orientation, anxiety, palpitations, and irritability.
St 36	Three Mile Point	Two chon down from the kneecap and four chon to the outside of the leg.	This point strength-ens and nourishes qi, relieves fatigue, and regulates energy flow. Calms and sharpens the mind.

Point Abbreviation	Name of Point	How You Find It	Benefits
Sp 2	Great Metropolis	On the inside of the foot at the large joint at the base of the big toe.	Regulates stomach and spleen qi, and calms restlessness.
Lv 3	Great Rushing	On the top side of the foot, go between the big and second toes; trace up the webbing between the metatarsal bones until the bones come together, forming a depression.	Regulates and tonifies the liver, regulating the smooth flow of qi. Reduces worry and stress related to decision making. Promotes relaxation.

This routine helps with mental relaxation and reduces unwanted thought patterns:

1. **Start with belly breathing, grounding, and centering (refer to Chapter 2).**

2. **Open your chest by stretching your arms back and rotating your hands back and forth.**

3. **Use bilateral holds and press GB 13 followed by GB 21 and St 13.**

   Use sustained pressure for the points that are empty, or pulsating pressure for the full points.

4. **Use all four fingers of each hand to hold the four spleen points — Sp 17, 18, 19, and 20 — simultaneously.**

   Use sustained pressure for one to three minutes.

5. **Use bilateral holds for K 27, St 36, Lv 3, and Sp 2.**

   Use sustained or alternating pressure as indicated.

6. **Relax by following your breath and listening to the sounds around you. Observe your body's sensations as you integrate the flow of qi.**

Anxiety-reducing pressure points

The points in this section are helpful in reducing anxiety, and we incorporate them in the routine later in this section. Study the points included in Table 8-4 and locate them in Figures 8-1 and 8-3.

Table 8-4		Acupoints for Reducing Anxiety	
Point Abbreviation	**Name of Point**	**How You Find It**	**Benefits**
HP 7	Great Mound	Go to the palm side of the wrist crease and find the point halfway between the inside and outside of the wrist.	Calms the spirit; used for mania, hysteria, insomnia, panic, fear, sadness, and weariness.
HP 6	Inner Gate	Palm side of the hand, in the middle of the arm, three finger-widths above the wrist crease.	Calms the spirit; used for palpitations, anxiety, and shock. Good for nausea.
TW 5	Outer Gate	Three fingers above the wrist crease on the outside of the hand.	Regulates qi flow through the meridian; can be used for excess fear.
H 7	Spirit Gate	Palm side up, go to the outer edge of the wrist, at the crease of the wrist under the little finger.	Used for anxiety, palpitations, fear, sighing, forgetfulness, mania, and depression.
H 5	Connecting Palace	Palm side of the hand, under the little finger, one chon above the wrist crease on the forearm.	Used for palpitations associated with fear, heart pounding, headache, anxiety, and fear of people.
Lu 1	Central Treasury	This point is located on your rib cage, one chon down from where your arm meets your chest wall. Use your thumbs and press this point toward the breastbone.	This point opens the chest and allows deeper breathing. It helps to balance and release stored emotions.
CV 17	Upper Sea of Qi	Go to the exact center of the breastbone, halfway between the top and bottom, and then drop slightly lower.	Used for calming and centering, nervousness, anxiety, and depression.

After reviewing the points in Table 8-4, put them into action in this routine, which helps ease anxiety woes:

1. **Prepare with belly breathing, grounding, and centering (refer to Chapter 2).**

2. **Place your hands together in prayer position and lift your elbows, holding for 30 seconds. Then stretch your arms backward, rotating your hands in both directions to create a good stretch.**

3. **Hold HP 7 on one side of the body, followed by HP 6 and TW 5 (you can hold these two together at the same time; they're opposite each other on the wrist).**

4. **Hold H 7 followed by H 5.**

5. **Repeat on the other arm.**

6. **Use bilateral holds for both Lu 1s.**

7. **End with CV 17.**

Worry-free reflexology

Reflexology can also be helpful in reducing the mental worry of worrywarts. The routine earlier in the chapter, "Reflexology to the stress rescue," focuses on emotional and physical stress. This routine deals with mental stress, the need to ease the mind of worry that goes round and round:

1. **Wash your feet, and then center and warm up.**

2. **Thumb-walk and use circular motions to detect and release any imbalances in the reflex areas on the foot for the stomach, spleen, heart, and small intestine (see Figure 8-6).**

3. **If you experience worry and anxiety in a specific part of your body, be sure to pay attention to the associated reflex areas.**

4. **End with thumb-walking and circular motions to the solar plexus and the adrenals, both of which generate and manage anxiety and worry.**

5. **Repeat with the other foot.**

6. **Spend some time relaxing and enjoying the benefits of your session. Relaxation allows the body to feel what it's like to be free of worry and anxiety.**

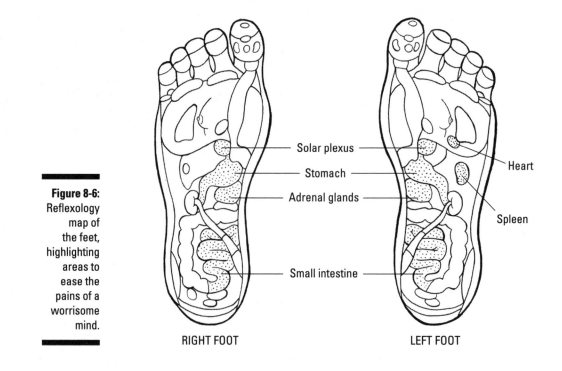

Figure 8-6:
Reflexology
map of
the feet,
highlighting
areas to
ease the
pains of a
worrisome
mind.

Solar plexus

Stomach

Adrenal glands

Heart

Spleen

Small intestine

RIGHT FOOT

LEFT FOOT

Don't Let Depression Keep You Down

Much as we'd like to, we're not going to tell you that you should try to live your life without ever feeling depressed. Going through life and never feeling a little down is impossible. When you suffer a loss, or can't express yourself in an important area of your life, you may get a bad case of the blues.

Depression is often seen as the opposite side of anger, or, as Freud said, anger turned against self. Anger itself is a symptom of being blocked in some aspect of your life. Maybe someone is breaching your boundaries, or you're trying to push the river, making something happen when its time hasn't yet come. Knowing the source of your emotions is the first step to allowing change.

People can be genetically predisposed to depression, so if this problem runs in your family, you need to be aware that you could be at risk of this condition. Females are especially susceptible to depression. According to the National Institute of Mental Health, women experience depression about twice as often as men.

Uplifting acupressure

In oriental medicine, depression and anger are imbalances in the liver and gall bladder meridians. As we discuss in Chapter 3, in Chinese medicine the liver meridian makes decisions, and the gall bladder meridian carries them out. Are you having trouble making decisions? Or do you feel frustrated making your dreams come true? Maybe you feel your life has no purpose, or you've lost connection to your heart. Take some time to connect with yourself, treating the acupoints in Table 8-5, shown earlier in the chapter in Figures 8-1, 8-2, and 8-3, by using the corresponding routine we provide in this section.

Table 8-5	Acupoints for Treating Depression		
Point Abbreviation	*Name of Point*	*How You Find It*	*Benefits*
Lv 3	Great Rushing	On the top side of the foot, go between the big and second toes; trace up the webbing between the metatarsal bones until the bones come together, forming a depression.	The source point rebalances the liver meridian, which assists the smooth flow of qi throughout the body. Provides an overall calming effect.
Lv 5	Draining Canal	Between the calf muscle and the tibia, in a small depression on the bone, five chon above the inner anklebone.	Eases depression, fear, and palpitations.
GB 20	Wind Pool	Along the ridge of your occipital bone halfway between your ear and spine; between the two muscles that come together.	Relieves irritability, and clears the mind.
GB 21	Shoulder Well	On the top of the shoulder, halfway between the point of your shoulder and the base of your neck. In the belly of the muscle.	Relieves frustration, irritability, and fatigue. Used for stiffness and pain of the neck, shoulder, and upper back.

(continued)

Table 8-5 *(continued)*

Point Abbreviation	Name of Point	How You Find It	Benefits
Lu 1	Central Treasury	This point is located on your rib cage, one chon down from where your arm meets your chest wall. Use your thumbs and press this point toward the breastbone.	This point opens the chest and allows deeper breathing. It helps to balance and release stored emotions.
K 27	Shu Mansion	Under the collarbone in the depression next to the breastbone.	Used for headaches due to mental strain, mental fatigue, dis-orientation, anxiety, palpitations, and irritability.
CV 17	Upper Sea of Qi	Go to the exact center of the breastbone, half-way between the top and bottom, and then drop slightly lower.	Used for calming and centering, ner-vousness, anxiety, and depression.
CV 14	Great Palace Gate	Two chon below the bottom of your breast-bone in the midline of the body; hold gently.	Used for palpitations and anxiety, hyste-ria, fear, insanity, and depression.

Use the following routine whenever you need a little emotional lift, or use it regularly to help alleviate depression:

1. **Prepare with breathing, grounding, centering, and stretching exercises (refer to Chapter 2).**

2. **Use bilateral holds on Lv 3, followed by Lv 5, GB 20, GB 21, Lu 1, and K 27.**

   Use sustained or alternating pressure as indicated.

3. **End by holding CV 17 with one hand while holding CV 14 with the other hand.**

4. **Give yourself time to lie still and familiarize yourself with the free-flowing qi.**

Easing the blues with reflexology

Reflexology can also help improve your mood and alleviate depression. If you're feeling low and enjoy practicing reflexology, try this routine:

1. **Start with foot washing, centering, and a warm up.**

2. **Use the reflex areas on the foot for the liver, gall bladder, and heart (see Figure 8-7).**

   Thumb-walk and use circular motions to detect and release any imbalances.

3. **Work the spine, shoulders, and neck areas.**

   Anger and depression are often expressed through tension in postural muscles, so pay particular attention to these areas if you're angry or depressed.

   As always, if you hold your emotions in a specific pattern, be sure to pay attention to the associated reflex areas.

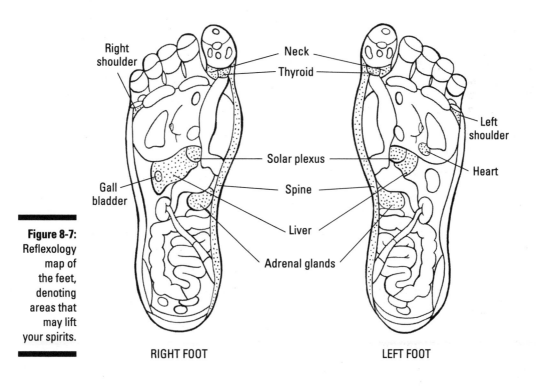

Figure 8-7:
Reflexology map of the feet, denoting areas that may lift your spirits.

RIGHT FOOT   LEFT FOOT

4. Use thumb-walking and circular motions on the adrenal and thyroid reflex areas as well as the solar plexus, which is a major site for stored anger.

5. Repeat with the other foot.

6. Allow yourself time to enjoy feeling more open and peaceful.

Part III

Where Does It Hurt? Treating Common Aches and Ailments

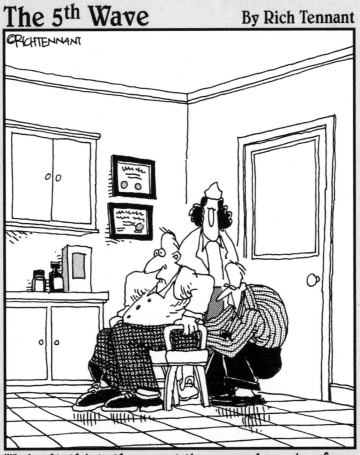

The 5th Wave   By Rich Tennant

"I don't think the crackling sound coming from your lower back is as serious as you thought. Just relax and I'll have this Rice Krispie Square out of your back pocket in no time."

In this part . . .

In Part III, we target specific areas of the body that may be causing you pain or problems. No matter what your most pressing issue, chances are good that you'll find helpful treatments for it in this part.

We start at the feet, work our way up the leg, and move into the hips. From aching heels to sore hamstrings, you find the keys to relief in this part. Backaches are a big problem for many people, so we address that in this part, as well. Having pain in your hands or arms? We have that covered, too. And if you have trouble in your stomach or chest areas, you'll want to zero in on those sections of this part. Then we head higher up, tackling headaches and problems related to the face.

You might say that this is "the part for all your parts."

Chapter 9

Putting Your Best Foot Forward

*N*o matter how big or small, all feet have one thing in common: For something that looks so simple, the foot is surprisingly complex. About 25 percent of all the bones in your body are found in your feet — along with more than 20 muscles, numerous tendons and ligaments, and assorted other anatomical bits and parts. In other words, your feet have lots of intricate — and often neglected and overworked — parts. So you're left with lots of places where pain can occur and really bring the entire operation to a screeching halt.

And because your feet have so many individual parts packed so closely together in a relatively small space, one small pain can quickly affect an increasingly larger area of your foot. In addition, your feet and ankles are the foundation upon which the entire rest of your body depends — they literally carry the weight of everything else in your anatomy. So, for example, if foot pain causes you to walk awkwardly or distribute your weight unevenly, you may wind up with pain in your legs and back.

Ankles are small compared to the rest of the body, and a lot of weight bears down on this rather narrow joint, so the joint has to be pretty strong to provide enough support. For this reason, it's important to nip the problem in the bud, addressing and alleviating foot and ankle pain at the very start.

Fortunately, we can give you hope. Acupressure can assist the movement of stagnant qi accumulating in the many joints of your feet and ankles, increasing flexibility and movement. But reflexology may be your first choice, because pressing, moving, and stimulating the feet directly relieves muscular tension as well as reflexively moving qi.

Identifying the Culprit

Before you can treat your foot pain, you need to figure out what's causing it in the first place. Removing the pain without treating the source is just like applying a temporary bandage — the pain will return. Lots of things — ranging from mild annoyances to major health concerns — can cause pain or discomfort in the foot and lower leg. In some cases the cause of the pain may not be resolvable — such as with damaged nerves from diabetes. In those cases you can still use acupressure and reflexology to ease the discomfort and slow the degeneration process.

Often, the cause of foot pain is blatantly obvious. If you spend ten straight hours on your feet at work while standing on an unforgiving concrete floor, you don't need the skills of Sherlock Holmes to figure out why your feet are in agony. In order for acupressure and reflexology to have a lasting effect, you need to find a solution to your working conditions. Same thing goes for pain that starts right after you suffer a broken toe — the pain will remain as the toe heals. But there's good news: These bodywork techniques will help the toe heal faster and reduce the pain of healing by encouraging the flow of nourishing qi.

Sometimes the root of your pain may be a bit more of a mystery. What if you have foot discomfort first thing in the morning, before you even take a single step? Or what about feet that never seem to feel better, no matter how long you soak them in that foot bath? In these cases, you need to proceed with caution until you have a diagnosis. You don't want the pressure you use to cause damage to already damaged tissue.

In this section, we cover both scenarios.

Recognizing common causes of pain

Several everyday scenarios commonly cause foot pain. Here, we discuss a few of the most likely culprits:

- **The strain of the daily grind:** Quite a few foot problems are caused by what amounts to wear and tear — you put a lot of miles on your feet and all that use is bound to take its toll. And, unfortunately, you really can't avoid putting a certain amount of miles on your feet — at least, not unless you plan to spend your entire life in bed. For city dwellers especially, walking considerable distances is simply an inevitable part of daily life. Then again, just standing still is tough on your feet — and in some ways, it's worse than walking because standing in one spot exerts continuous pressure on the same limited group of muscles, causing increasing fatigue.

In addition, if you stand on your feet all day, your veins can get weak, allowing fluid to build up in the ankles. This fluid build-up is called *edema* and can increase joint stiffness. Acupressure can stimulate venous return and lymph flow, so the ankle routine later in this chapter can be very helpful for alleviating fluid build-up, too.

✔ **Fashionable yet painful shoes:** Perhaps you mistreat your feet by subjecting them to tasks and conditions that they were never designed to endure. Stiletto heels and pointy toes, anyone? High heels are often blamed for ankle problems, but other types of shoes (such as clogs) can also put strain on the feet and ankles. When you decide to suffer for the sake of fashion, your feet often pay the price. (Not surprisingly, women are several times more likely than men to experience foot problems.)

According to the American Podiatric Medical Association, heels over two inches high change the way a woman normally walks, and heels over three inches put seven times the pressure on the ball of the foot! In addition, the small of your back suffers with the change in body positioning.

✔ **Corns and bunions:** These annoying foot problems are another cause of discomfort. They can both be caused by a change in weight distribution as you walk, but having corns changes how you walk even more, causing misalignment and pain in the bones and joints.

✔ **Hobbies and such:** Certain lifestyle habits can be tough on your feet. If you do a lot of hiking or climbing (even if it's climbing a lot of stairs), you're causing a lot of stress for your feet.

✔ **The way you sit:** If you often sit with your feet crossed or tucked underneath you, you can cause a lot of strain and stress on your feet, especially over extended periods of time.

✔ **Accidents and injuries:** Feet tend to be unlucky, because they're often in the wrong place at the wrong time — or they're forced to suffer the consequences of their owner's clumsiness and carelessness. As a result, feet endure more broken bones, sprains, twisted ankles, and stubbed toes than anyone can count.

An added complication is that foot injuries can heal slowly or incorrectly because people with these types of injuries are frequently unable or unwilling to stay off their feet long enough to allow for proper recovery.

Foot problems are extremely common. A study conducted by the American Podiatric Medical Association (APMA) in 2004 found that 31 percent of those interviewed had foot or ankle problems within a year's time.

Finding a mysterious source of pain

The cause of your foot pain is often blatantly obvious. When the origins of your foot pain aren't so clear, though, you need to spend a bit of time evaluating your health and family history. Here are a few causes that you may not have considered:

- ✔ **Hereditary conditions:** Sometimes people are born with conditions that cause foot pain, including things like flat feet or high arches.

- ✔ **General health problems:** People with diabetes and circulatory conditions also frequently experience pain in their feet. (People who suffer from these conditions should make their doctor aware of any new or increased foot pain, in case it signifies a serious problem.)

- ✔ **Bone spurs:** Bone spurs are growths that develop along the edges of bones and can cause pain by rubbing against nearby nerves and other bones. They generally occur with aging but also can be caused by various medical conditions, such as osteoarthritis and plantar fasciitis.

- ✔ **Hammertoes:** Hammertoes are toes in which the middle joint sticks out, producing a painful "buckling" effect, which is often complicated by the growth of a corn in that area.

Daily tips for easing foot pain (aside from bodywork)

Obviously, you can't change the shape (or size) of the feet you were born with, but you can take several steps to make those feet more comfortable:

- ✔ Arch supports can be helpful in treating a variety of foot problems, including flat feet. In severe cases, you may need to order a custom-fitted support from your podiatrist, but generally an over-the-counter support will work just fine.

- ✔ Cushioned shoe inserts can often make a big difference in how your feet feel at the end of the day, especially if you walk a lot.

Look for insoles with gel cushioning, which many people say work the best. If you have flat feet or fallen arches, arch supports can also help.

- ✔ Exercise and stretching can relax the foot muscles — particularly those around the ankles — which can make a big difference in your comfort level.

- ✔ Pain creams and over-the-counter pain relievers can often provide temporary relief, but it's not a good idea to rely on these (especially medications) for extended periods of time.

Obviously, you can't do much to change the conditions you were born with (although medical treatment may be able to help with some conditions to a certain extent). In these cases, often the best you can do is to try the following:

✔ Keep your feet in the best shape possible by treating them to regular preventative-maintenance therapy sessions.

✔ Promptly address any specific problems and pain that you have.

If you're facing pains you weren't born with but have developed over time, ask your doctor for recommendations on treating them and check out our advice in the nearby sidebar "Daily tips for easing foot pain (aside from bodywork)."

Relieving Pain in Your Kickers

The following routines are great for reducing ankle pain, swelling, and stiffness as well as foot pain and discomfort. They can also promote healing from sprains and strains, which is important because improper healing from ankle injuries may leave you with a weak joint. Weakness in the ankles translates into stress on the knees and hips, leading to pain in these joints as well.

Obviously, these routines are limited when you're trying to help "surface problems" like blisters and corns (in those cases, your best bet is to also use topical treatments like ointments and creams specifically for those ailments). Still, by reducing your pain and making your feet more comfortable, these exercises can greatly improve your overall foot health. When poor foot alignment causes corns, stretching can be beneficial along with evaluating and correcting the biomechanics of your gait. This treatment requires the professional help of a physical therapist, orthopedist, or doctor of physical medicine.

Ankles and feet: Pressure on the acupoints for fast relief

The main points you use in this section are ankle and feet points on the kidney, bladder, stomach, spleen, and gall bladder meridians. Moving blocks in the ankles opens pathways for stagnant qi to move out of the feet as well. We show you the points (see Figures 9-1 and 9-2) and then make suggestions on how to use them.

Keep in mind that every point has multiple functions, and we use the same point to do different things in different treatments. Table 9-1 gives you information on the points and their benefits (if you aren't familiar with the measurement term *chon,* see Chapter 3). You can provide benefit to any foot or ankle problem by using the points in Table 9-1 — we recommend using them all for overall ankle and foot well-being, but if you don't have time, just work on the points that address the specific conditions we identify in the table.

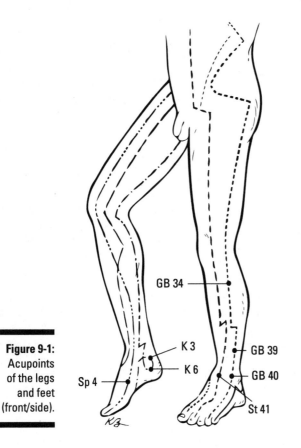

Figure 9-1:
Acupoints
of the legs
and feet
(front/side).

GB 34

K 3

K 6

Sp 4

GB 39

GB 40

St 41

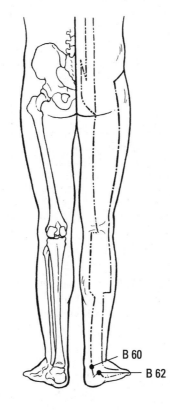

Figure 9-2:
Acupoints of
the legs and
feet (back).

B 60

B 62

Table 9-1	Pain-Relieving Points for the Ankles and Feet		
Point Abbreviation	*Name of Point*	*How You Find It*	*Benefits*
K 3	Great Ravine	Halfway between the Achilles tendon and the inside anklebone.	Reduces swelling and pain. Strengthens the kidney meridian, which governs legs and bones.
K 6	Shining Sea	One chon below inside anklebone.	Relieves swelling, and relieves heel and ankle pain.
St 41	Stream Divide	Middle of the foot in front of the anklebone.	Used for the symptoms of ankle pain, sprain, or drop foot. Reduces heat and inflammation.
B 60	Kunlun Mountains	Halfway between the Achilles tendon and the outer anklebone.	Relaxes tendons. Increases qi flow to the legs and ankles. Reduces ankle and heel pain. Can be useful in arthritis in the ankle.
B 62	Extending Vessel	One and a half chon below the outer anklebone in the indentation.	Relaxes tendons and muscles.
GB 34	Yang Mound	In the depression below and slightly in front of the head of the fibula (outer leg bone).	Sends qi to tendons and ligaments. Use for weakness and to reduce inflammation.
GB 39	Suspended Bell	Three chon (one hand-width) above the outer anklebone on the back edge of the fibula, or outer leg bone.	Increases qi and blood flow to the leg.

Point Abbreviation	Name of Point	How You Find It	Benefits
GB 40	Hill Ruins	Directly in front of the outer anklebone in the hollow.	Promotes healing for ankle sprains and strain.
Sp 4	Grandfather-Grandson	On the inside of the foot, one chon behind the base of the big toe. Find the bone in the arch of the foot, hook your finger into the arch from underneath, and press upward.	Stimulates the movement of leg qi, and releases tension in the arch of the foot.

Here's an exercise that can help ankles and feet feel their best:

1. **Start with deep belly breathing, grounding, and centering (refer to Chapter 2).**

2. **Stretch the ankle by doing the following:**

   - Rotating it in a circle, first clockwise and then counterclockwise.

   - Sitting on the floor or bed with an outstretched leg. Flex your foot and reach forward to grab your toes. If you can't reach your toes, take a towel and loop it around your foot, holding onto the ends so that you have a sling around your foot. Slowly lean back to create a gentle stretch on the ankle. If you have an injury, be very gentle; never cause pain. You can even omit the stretches altogether if you need to.

   - If you're working on someone else, gently do these stretches for her. Make sure she doesn't help when you put her ankle through its range of motion. Be very cautious if your friend has an injury — you may want to omit the stretches altogether.

3. **For overall wellness, alternately press and release each point in Table 9-1, focusing attention on the sore points — if you're pressed for time, skip ahead to Step 4.**

   Disperse points that seem very full or stagnant by pulsing your pressure. Tonify or build qi in empty points by holding sustained pressure until the acupoint fills up.

If you have active inflammation, be sure to use light pressure on inflamed areas. If you have an ankle injury, press the points above and below the injury to encourage qi flow through the injured area. You may want to do this every day until your ankle is healed.

4. **If you're pressed for time or just want to focus on a particular issue, focus on these key points:**

   - **Swollen ankle:** K 3, K 6, St 41, Sp 4

   - **Sprained ankle:** K 3, K 6, St 41, GB 34, GB 40

   - **Fallen arches:** GB 39, Sp 4

   - **Plantar fasciitis:** St 41, B 60, B 62, Sp 4

   - **Arthritis:** K 3, K 6, St 41, B 60, B 62

5. **Enjoy your well-earned 5 to 10 minutes of relaxation. Focus on nothing at all except your breath and the warmth in your relaxed yet stimulated feet.**

Reflexology: Rotate, roll, and rub away!

Reflexology can be helpful in treating injuries and in reducing swelling in feet and ankles. Co-author Synthia has seen swelling reduce by as much as 25 percent after a session when stimulating the lymphatic pathways. The lymph system drains excess fluid from an area, helping with swelling from standing on your feet all day or inflammation swelling from an injury. Reflexology is especially helpful when the ankle itself is too painful to work on directly. In addition to assisting the body in healing after injuries, it can improve qi flow through the area, reducing stagnation, pain, and stiffness.

Here's a routine that can be helpful:

1. **Sit in a comfortable chair and put your foot in your lap.**

   If you can't comfortably put your foot in your lap, use a reflexology tool. Try a tennis ball in a sock or any reflexology tool you have (see Chapter 2 for more on these tools).

2. **Follow your warm-up routine of foot washing, belly breathing, foot rolling, and foot stripping.**

3. **Use your thumbs to "thumb-walk" all over the end of the heel in the foot reflex area.**

4. **Finger- or thumb-walk up the lymphatic strip (see Figure 9-3), starting at the heel and walking toward the toe.**

   Do this step several times, starting each time at the heel and moving toward the toe.

5. **Use your thumbs to do circular motions on the heel area (reflex areas for the feet, ankles, and sciatic nerve) and the lymphatic strip.**

   Finding the ankle points may be difficult, because the ankle has no designation on the map. Generally, ankles are considered part of the reflex area for the feet found on the very small wedge on the end of both heels.

   Take extra time where you feel soreness, stickiness, or crystals.

6. **End by thumb-walking several times up and down the lymphatic strip.**

7. **If you're using a tool, put it on the floor under your foot and simply roll your foot over the tool along the reflex areas, stopping when you feel soreness and working that area thoroughly.**

   Use as much pressure as is comfortable.

8. **Repeat with the other foot (although you can skip this step if you're assisting an injury on one foot only).**

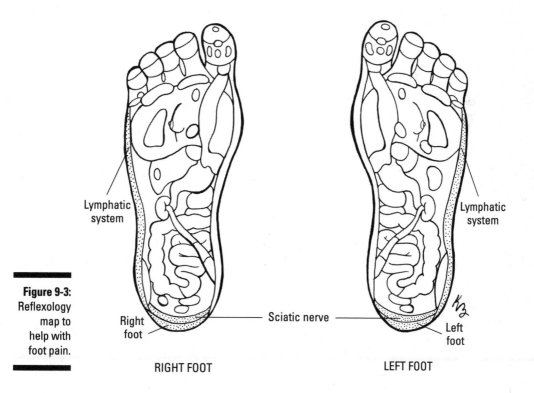

Figure 9-3:
Reflexology
map to
help with
foot pain.

Lymphatic system

Lymphatic system

Right foot

Sciatic nerve

Left foot

RIGHT FOOT

LEFT FOOT

Chapter 10

Healing the Leg and Hip Regions

*I*f feet are the foundation of the body (see Chapter 9), legs and hips are the load-bearing walls that keep it standing upright and properly supported. Think about it: Every time the foot takes a step, the leg is right there taking the trip along with it.

In this chapter, we discuss some of the most common hip and leg problems, and we demonstrate bodywork techniques that can help you address — and hopefully correct — any imbalances that may be causing or worsening the pain. By making sure your energy flow is in sync, you can also put your system in optimum condition to recover from any illness or injury that may be bringing you pain.

Common Leg Ailments

Legs really get a workout through the entire day. Whether you're walking, standing, driving, dancing, or doing any of the other activities you do on a daily basis, your legs are bearing at least a moderate amount of stress or strain. And don't forget lifting. By now, everyone's heard the advice to "lift with your legs, not your back." Well, that's great for your back — but not so great for your poor legs.

Hips and knees face their share of problems and challenges, too. In order for you to be able to move in all directions, your hips need to have a very large range of motion. And the hardest job for any joint is to provide great stability with a lot of movement — they're sort of opposite needs. No wonder hips get tired and sore. Pain and stiffness in the hips (which can often increase with age) can make if difficult to do everyday tasks — or even to move much at all.

And although the knee seems like a simple joint, it's actually a masterful balance of opposing forces that align and propel movement. Of course, with lots of different forces, you expect lots of different problems. No surprise, knees are the site of common complaints both for athletes and for less active people.

In the following list, we touch on a few of the most common leg ailments, all of which can be treated with acupressure and reflexology (in addition to medical treatment when appropriate, of course):

✔ **Muscle cramps and injuries:** People often experience leg pain as a result of muscle cramps. Often felt in the calves or upper thighs, muscle cramps can strike during or after exercise or other physical exertion. Muscles are also susceptible to injuries as a result of accidents or overexertion. Anyone who's suffered a torn or strained muscle knows how painful those injuries can be. Reflexology and acupressure move qi through these sore areas, relieving stagnation, increasing nourishment, and improving circulation to the tissue.

Dehydration can cause or worsen muscle cramps in the legs. Be sure to stay properly hydrated, especially during and after exercise.

✔ **Knee problems:** Knee problems can be incredibly painful and debilitating. Unfortunately, they're also fairly common — especially for people who are very active or athletic. Most types of sports and other athletic activities involve at least a moderate amount of strain on the knees. Anyone who follows sports knows how often athletes are sidelined by various knee problems. Increasing nourishing qi can help the body's healing efforts, speeding recovery time and ensuring the most complete healing process possible.

✔ **Vein-related conditions:** Many of the most common (and most serious) health problems occurring in the legs involve the veins. Veins are vessels that carry blood to the heart. (Then there are arteries, of course, which bring blood from the heart to the rest of the body.) About two-thirds of the body's blood supply is carried via the veins. Acupressure and reflexology have a direct impact on circulation: where qi goes, blood follows. The healing arts are ideal for assisting the body with some types of circulatory conditions; always use caution if serious conditions are suspected, and never use pressure directly on a sore vein. Two conditions in particular affect a significant number of people:

• **Varicose veins** are probably the most well-known vein-related problem in the legs. This is a condition in which veins become swollen and enlarged. Typically, this condition is associated with large blue veins that protrude through the skin of the legs. The majority of cases of varicose veins occur in women. Heredity plays a role, although women are generally at greater risk during and after pregnancy.

Varicose veins aren't just a cosmetic problem. They can interfere with proper blood flow and cause circulation problems. Acupressure and reflexology are ideal for assisting with the circulation of qi and blood. Take care not to press on a varicosity; use only light contact with no pressure on any points that are directly on top of a vein that's enlarged, swollen, or painful.

- **Deep vein thrombosis (DVT)** is a condition in which a blood clot forms deep within a vein in the leg or pelvic region. Although this condition can cause cramping and circulation problems, the more serious risk is that the blood clot will break off and travel to the lung — which can be deadly. People who spend prolonged periods of time sitting (especially in cramped conditions) or lying in bed are at greater risk of developing DVT. This is a serious and potentially deadly condition that shouldn't be treated with acupressure. Pressure on the clot can release it into circulation. Only the professionally trained should work with this condition. Reflexology can be used more safely as long as the person is under medical care and supervision.

- **Restless leg syndrome (RLS):** This common leg-related problem affects up to 10 percent of the population at some point in their lives. Although not deadly, this condition can still be very painful and disruptive to the people who suffer from it, especially if they have a severe case. The primary symptoms of RLS are a compulsive urge to move your legs and a strange sensation — often described as a "creepy crawly" feeling — up and down the legs. These symptoms occur most often and most severely when you're lying down. As a result, getting a good night's sleep can be nearly impossible for people with RLS. In Chinese medicine, RLS is considered a condition that can be addressed by directing unruly qi and smoothing qi flow. This can be done with acupressure and reflexology. If you go to a professional, he or she may use Chinese herbs as well.

Caffeine, chocolate, and alcohol frequently worsen the symptoms of RLS. Likewise, certain prescription medications (such as those used to treat high blood pressure and depression) can also sometimes increase the severity of symptoms. If you suffer from RLS, ask your doctor for advice on which substances you should avoid.

Addressing the Source of Pain

Knowing the source of your pain helps determine where you focus your sessions. For example, if your hip pain is because of poor mechanics of the feet, your session will include the feet and hips. The bottom line, however, is that your body has its own healing plans underway. Bringing qi into the area gives the body more to work with and provides assistance and support.

Several factors can contribute to pain in the leg and hip — or worsen any pain that already exists:

- ✔ **Age:** With age, the risk of suffering a serious hip injury as a result of even a "minor" fall increases. The healing powers of the body also weaken as you age, making the addition of healing qi a welcomed support.

- ✔ **Physical activity:** If you're very active (especially if you suddenly become much more active than you were previously), you can put strain on your legs and hips until your body becomes accustomed to this new level of physical activity. On the other hand, if you're very inactive, you can also develop strains due to lack of movement and muscle weakening. Lack of movement promotes conditions of stagnant qi, such as arthritis and adhesions. Tonifying techniques can be helpful in these conditions.

- ✔ **Accidents or injuries:** Many leg problems are the result of accidents. Examples include the broken leg suffered after a skier attempted a really challenging trail, and the fracture caused by slipping on a patch of ice. These types of injuries require medical treatment and a necessary recovery period. Speed and completeness of recovery depend on adequate qi levels. Your acupressure and reflexology skills will be well used here.

- ✔ **Health conditions:** Many conditions can cause pain in the hips and legs, including arthritis, lupus, diabetes, sprains, fractures, and lots more. In this case, you need to know the underlying cause to make significant improvements. Bodywork on the hips and legs in this case will be temporarily relieving, but you need to address the underlying cause to get a more lasting effect.

- ✔ **Genetic conditions:** Examples of genetic conditions include muscular dystrophy and congenital deformities. In these cases, bodywork can be useful to decrease discomfort.

- ✔ **Lifestyle factors:** Participating in many athletic activities, for example, can increase your risk for leg and hip problems.

- ✔ **Certain medications:** Some medications can increase the likelihood of leg cramps, swelling, and other painful conditions. Knowing what medications your receiver is taking is important to avoid unwanted interactions. For example, because bodywork lowers blood pressure, a healing session can have an accumulative, synergistic effect on someone taking medication to lower his or her blood pressure.

Sometimes, tracking down the cause of your hip and leg pain is a challenge. Of course, if you've suffered a broken leg, the cause of your pain is blatantly obvious. On the other hand, if you're plagued by a gradually worsening pain in the lower leg, you may have a tougher time tracking the roots of that problem. When you're trying to determine the cause of leg pain, keep the following in mind:

✔ **Most hip problems** are caused by one of three things: a fall or other injury, a chronic medical problem (such as arthritis), or poor bio-mechanics from issues of foot, knee, or pelvis alignment.

Because the hips and legs are part of such a complex system of muscles, bones, joints, ligaments, and other body parts, a problem that originates in one limited area of the body can quickly start affecting the rest of this larger region.

✔ **Most knee problems** originate in either the hips or the ankles and feet, unless you suffer a direct trauma, like getting hit in the knee with a ball or twisting your knee in a fall.

If you're an athlete, you may have knee problems from overuse, from pivoting motions, or from *repetitive use* — doing the same thing over and over. If you're not an athlete, you may have knee problems from muscular imbalance that pulls your knee out of proper alignment. In either case, when helping ease the discomfort of knee problems, be sure to work the ankle and hip as well.

Naturally, you want to make your doctor aware of any sudden or severe pain that you may be experiencing; he or she may be able to help diagnose the problem and the cause.

Healing Routines for the Knees, Hips, and Legs

When practicing bodywork, your best strategy is to look at any complicating factors you may have, and try to adjust or address those that are under your control. Treat the underlying causes if you know what they are. Because acupressure and reflexology don't actually treat diseases or conditions, you're treating imbalances of qi. As qi flow becomes more even, the body has access to its unique healing properties and can maximize its healing efforts. Ask yourself what feels empty and what feels full. See Chapter 4 for more information if needed.

Obviously, you must have realistic expectations. For example, bodywork alone can't magically make a broken bone whole again. On the other hand, adjusting imbalances in your energy flow may help reduce the pain you feel from circulation problems by encouraging proper blood flow. Just how effective healing therapy can be varies greatly depending on the type and severity of the problem causing your pain.

Getting a leg up with acupressure

Here's a healing routine to use for knees and hips. The meridians you use are mostly the gall bladder, bladder, stomach, and spleen. Basically, these points promote qi flow through the entire leg, so you can use them for any leg ailment you have. They're great to relieve bursitis, tendonitis, or strains and sprains. You can use them to support healing, to promote recovery after a road race or athletic event, or simply to relieve the aches and pains from standing all day. You can work the acupoints of both joints for a full routine or work only the points for the joint you want to emphasize. As always, don't work directly on an injury, and be sure to get proper medical help for any problems you have. You can find these points in Tables 10-1 and 10-2 and in Figures 10-1 and 10-2.

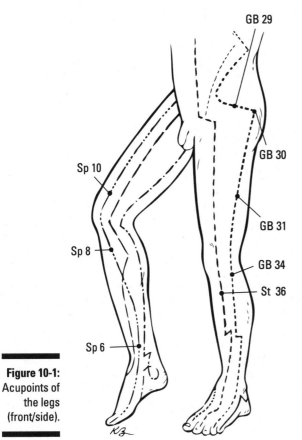

Figure 10-1:
Acupoints of the legs (front/side).

The legend of stomach 36

There's an interesting legend about the stomach 36 acupoint. According to the story, a general in an ancient Chinese army needed his troops to march a long distance to reach their destination. They were all tired from fighting and marching for so many weeks. At some point, the army stopped marching — they felt they couldn't go any farther. The general ordered his army doctor to use acupuncture on the stomach 36 point on every soldier. Legend has it that the troops marched for another 3 miles and reached their destination. From that day on, the point was called Three Mile Point.

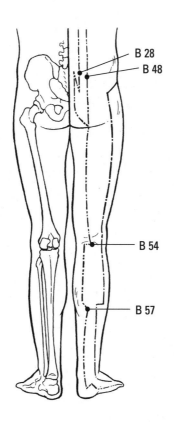

Figure 10-2:
Acupoints of
the legs and
low back
(back).

B 28
B 48
B 54
B 57

If you're reading through Tables 10-1 and 10-2, and you're not sure how to measure *chon*, flip to Chapter 3 for details.

Table 10-1	Acupoints of the Hip and Pelvis		
Point Abbreviation	**Name of Point**	**How You Find It**	**Benefits**
GB 29	Squatting Bone Hole	Place your hands on your hips, and then rotate your wrists so that your fingers are pointing downward. Bend your middle finger and it will fall just about on this point, which is one to two chon above the hipbone in the hip joint. It's easy to find if you squat and place your thumb in the midline of your side, right in the crease made by your leg.	Helps with inflammation in the hip joint; relieves muscle sprains and pain; used for sciatica; reduces muscle spasms in the thigh; relieves lower abdominal and lower back pain.
GB 30	Jumping Round	Divide the sacrum in half from top to bottom. Find the edge of the sacrum with your thumbs, and slide three-quarters of the way into the gluteal muscles from the middle of the sacrum.	Reduces hip joint inflammation; relieves muscle sprains, pain, and spasms, especially in the buttocks; used for sciatica; relieves lower abdominal and lower back pain.
GB 31	Wind Market	Find this point on the side of your thigh, halfway between your hipbone and knee. If you drop your arm alongside your leg, your middle finger should be right there. Be careful; it can be really tender.	Used for weakness in the thigh and knee; improves leg qi; used for lower back pain and sciatica.

Point Abbreviation	Name of Point	How You Find It	Benefits
GB 34	Yang Mound	This point is on the side of the leg, below your knee, slightly in front of the head of the outer leg bone (fibula).	Stimulates leg qi; strengthens weak extremities; relieves spasms and sciatica; reduces pain and inflammation in the hip and knee.
B 28	Bladder Shu	Two chon to either side of the spine, level with the fifth lumbar vertebrae.	Used for lower and sacral back pain and sciatica.
B 48 (May be numbered Bladder 54 on some meridian charts)	Bladder Vitals	Three chon to the side of the sacrum in the middle of the gluteal muscles of the buttocks. Very tender point.	Used for buttock, sacral, and lower back pain, and sciatica.

Table 10-2	Acupoints of the Knee		
Point Abbreviation	Name of Point	How You Find It	Benefits
B 54 (May be numbered as B 40 on some meridian charts)	Middle Crook	Right in the middle of the crease in the back of the knee.	Releases low back pain, stiffness, and tension; used for sciatica and herniated discs; moves qi through the knee, reducing muscle spasms, knee pain, and stiffness.
B 57	Supporting Mountain	In the back of the calf, one-third of the way between the knee and the ankle where the calf muscle splits.	Reduces muscle spasms in the calf; relieves cramps.

(continued)

Table 10-2 *(continued)*

Point Abbreviation	Name of Point	How You Find It	Benefits
St 36	Three Mile Point	One chon out from the shinbone and three chon below the patella (one palm width).	Used for general weakness, fatigue, and exhaustion. Stimulates leg qi and improves endurance. Often called "three more miles" — the amount of additional miles you can walk after stimulating it.
Sp 10	Sea of Blood	Three chon above the kneecap on the inside of the leg.	Moves qi through the leg.
Sp 8	Earth's Crux	Three chon down from the tibial tuberosity on the inside of the tibia (approximately one hand-width down from the patella).	Alleviates lower back pain and knee stiffness and pain.
Sp 6*	Three Yin Crossing	Three finger-widths above the inner ankle-bone along the back of the tibia.	This point has many functions and is also the crossing point of three major yin meridians of the leg. Useful for mobilizing leg qi.

* Never use this point during pregnancy.

Here's a routine that's often helpful for the legs, knees, and hips. Because the joints in the legs and hips all affect each other, do all the sequences in Step 3 if possible. If you don't have time, however, you can use specific sequences we highlight there for the areas you want to balance.

   1. Do your belly breathing while grounding and centering yourself (refer to Chapter 2).

2. Stretch your hamstrings (back of the leg), quadriceps (front of the leg), and the inside of your leg.

If you have a favorite stretch for these areas, use them. If you don't, here are some ideas (Hold each stretch for a minimum of 20 seconds and repeat each three times for the full effect.):

- Sit on the floor with both legs stretched out in front of you. Lift your arms over your head and bend forward, over your outstretched legs. Try to keep your back straight and lean out over your leg rather than folding your upper body. You can assist the stretch by grasping your toes with your hands. If you can't reach, use a towel; hold both ends and make a sling around your feet.

- Stretch the inside of your legs by sitting with your legs outstretched and opened as wide as you can. Take your arms over your head and lean forward as far as you comfortably can between your open legs. Keep your back straight. You can push your hips out behind you to get a better stretch on your inner thighs.

- To stretch the quadriceps, lie on your side. Flex the knee of your top leg, moving your foot to your buttocks. Reach back and grasp your ankle, pulling it toward your buttocks to improve the stretch. Repeat on the other side.

3. Using the bilateral approach or working one meridian at a time — balance the points by using sustained pressure to tonify the empty points or pulsating pressure to disperse the full points (refer to Chapter 4) — follow these sequences:

- **To address problems in the hip joints and buttocks as well as problems with the outside of the knee,** such as lateral collateral ligament (LCL) strains, hold GB 29 or 30 (whichever is more sore); press and release GB 31 and 34. This set of points is geared to the buttocks, pelvis, and the outside of the thigh.

- **To focus on the low back and sacrum (which affect the hips and legs and vice versa) and/or to relieve pain at the back of the knee,** hold B 28; press and release B 48, B 54, and B 57.

Always remember to treat the back of the knee with care and use light pressure on B 54.

- **To address the inside of the leg and knee and ease medial knee problems, such as sprains in the medial collateral ligament (MCL),** hold St 36; press and release Sp 6, Sp 8, and Sp 10.

4. End the session by lying quietly on your back, or sitting comfortably in a chair, with one hand on your lower abdomen and one hand on your solar plexus.

Relax and allow the benefits of the session to sink in.

Dancing to the beat of a different reflexology routine

This reflexology routine helps alleviate pain in the hips and knees:

1. **Start by washing and drying your feet.**

2. **If you haven't already stretched and performed deep breathing exercises, do some deep belly breathing now.**

3. **Sit in a chair or on a bed and cross your leg so that you can hold your foot in your lap.**

4. **Warm, stretch, and open your feet by first rolling your foot back and forth in your hand, and then stripping your foot from top to bottom (see Chapter 4 for an explanation of this technique).**

   Repeat three or four times to reduce restrictions.

5. **Wrap your middle fingers over the top of your foot and place your thumbs on the sole of your foot. Gently push your foot up into dorsiflexion (toes up), and then pull it down into plantar flexion (toes down).**

   Repeat this motion several times, rhythmically pumping your foot. This stimulates the reflex points along the top of the ankle and moves qi.

6. **Move your thumbs down to your heel and do thumb-walking along the reflex points for hips, sciatica, and knees (see Figure 10-3).**

   - If any spots are sore, use circular motions to work them out.
   - If any joints are inflamed, be sure to thumb-walk up the lymphatic strip along the outside of the foot, followed by circular motions on sore areas.

7. **Do circular motions on the reflex area for the adrenal glands to work out any sluggishness.**

   Stimulating the adrenal glands also promotes healing; the reflex points for the adrenal glands are located on the inside of the arch of the foot.

8. **Repeat with the other foot.**

9. **Relax.**

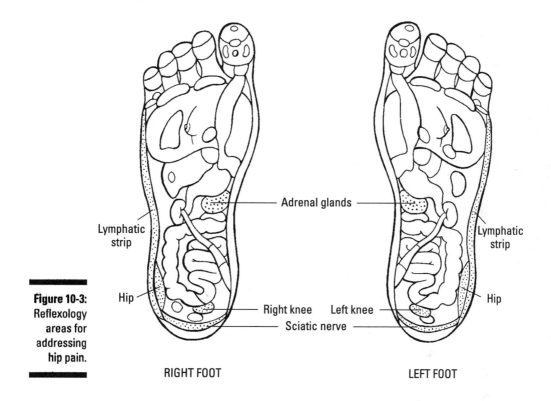

Figure 10-3:
Reflexology
areas for
addressing
hip pain.

Adrenal glands

Lymphatic
strip

Lymphatic
strip

Hip

Hip

Right knee   Left knee

Sciatic nerve

RIGHT FOOT   LEFT FOOT

Chapter 11

Relieving Backaches

*F*ortunately for most people, back pain is usually a temporary, limited-time thing, often brought on by strenuous activity or overexertion. Some unlucky souls, however, must cope with back pain constantly. This can make every day seem like an endless struggle with pain and tension in the back. Depending on the specific type of back problem, you may have difficulty doing even the simplest things, like sitting down or lying down in bed.

Many people are relieved to discover how effective acupressure and reflexology can be in reducing or eliminating their back pain. In this chapter, we help you figure out the source of your back pain so that you can apply acupressure safely and use the most effective points. Some causes of pain, like muscle tension, respond well to good stretching and deep pressure on the involved acupoints. Other causes, such as a herniated disc, require gentle stretching and less pressure. In all cases, acupressure and reflexology are great tools for back care. Use them together or individually to reduce the pain of muscle tension, aid the recovery of torn muscles or injured discs, reduce the stiffness of arthritis, relieve pressure on compressed nerves, and reduce or even eliminate pain. In this chapter, we explain just how the healing arts can help, and we provide a few healing routines to nip your pain in the bud (or at least give you a bit of relief!).

Understanding the Origins of Back Pain

"Back pain" is kind of a catchall term for pain, discomfort, or tenderness anywhere in the spinal region, or even sometimes in the hips, neck, and shoulders. In this chapter, though, we focus specifically on pain in the spinal area. We focus on other regions (hips, neck, and so on) in other parts of this book so that we can help you zero in on the techniques that will best target your particular pain.

Because the back takes up such a large part of your body, it makes sense that many specific types of problems can cause problems in this region. The following list outlines those specific types of problems:

- **Accidents and injuries:** In some cases, you may be able to pinpoint the exact moment your back began hurting. In these cases, tracing the cause of the pain may be easy. For example, if you begin experiencing pain in your upper back immediately after a strenuous basketball game, the reason for your pain is pretty obvious. On the other hand, sometimes the event that appears to cause the pain is really just a "precipitating incident," the final straw that breaks the camel's back. In this case, you usually have an underlying problem. Underlying problems can lie dormant for long periods of time until a little extra exertion reveals their presence. The extra exertion doesn't have to be too much; bending down to pick up a sock, falling asleep on a soft couch, or opening a sticking sliding door.

- **Impairments or abnormalities in the back:** Sometimes you don't need to look very far to find the root of your back pain. Some common causes of back pain include pinched nerves, herniated or ruptured disks, arthritis, muscle spasms, and abnormal curvature of the back.

  With these types of conditions, a doctor is often able to diagnose the problem through a variety of tests, possibly including an MRI or a CAT scan. The doctor may then be able to recommend a treatment plan that may help alleviate some of your pain. In severe cases, surgery may be necessary. (Fortunately, back pain rarely requires such extreme measures.) However, trying acupressure and reflexology while you're pursuing your treatment plan can be beneficial in relieving pain.

- **Problems in other areas of the body:** In some cases, the source of your back pain may not be quite so obvious. And for good reason — the pain may not actually be originating in your back at all. Organ dysfunction often refers pain into the back. For example, gall bladder and liver problems refer pain between the right shoulder blade and spine in the rhomboid muscles. Bladder trouble can refer into the sacral iliac joint, and pancreas issues can refer into the left mid and upper back. According to the basic principles of acupressure and reflexology, you may be feeling pain in one area of your body and it can travel along the meridian to another area. If you suspect organ dysfunction as the cause of your back pain, get a medical diagnosis before using alternative techniques. When you know what the problem is and are receiving proper treatment and care, you can use acupressure and reflexology to relieve discomfort and assist energy flow through the problem area.

If you don't have an injury or illness that could be affecting your back and you're trying to figure out what's causing your back pain, think about where — and how — you sit. Spending long periods of time on a hard chair or bench can frequently trigger backaches. Poor biomechanics in your workstation, poor posture, shoes, and repetitive actions can all contribute to your discomfort. Also, if you often have large and/or bulky items in your back pockets (a wallet, tools, and so on), they can cause you to sit unevenly, or sitting on them can compress the piriformis muscle causing sciatica and pain. Although acupressure and reflexology can help, the benefits won't last until the cause is removed.

Treating Your Aching Back

The bladder meridian is your highway to heaven if you experience back pain, because it's the main meridian flowing through your back. It begins at the inside of the orbit of your eye, travels over the top of your head, and down your back and legs to the outside of your little toe. It's the longest meridian in your body and takes a few strange curves along its path. For instance, when the bladder meridian reaches the base of your neck, it splits in two, sending two branches down each side of the back. The branches track the big muscle group, the erector spinae, that runs next to your spine and helps keep your back straight. One branch of the bladder meridian travels on the inside of this muscle group, between the muscle and your spine; the other branch travels on the outside of this muscle group. Not surprisingly, they're called the inner and outer branches of the bladder meridian.

Okay, we can just about manage a split in the line, but here's the rub: Different systems number the lines differently! Some systems number the inside line and then go down the leg to the knee before coming back up to get the outside line. Other systems, like the one we use, number the inside line, and then the outside line, and then travel down the leg. It doesn't really matter to the routines you're doing, but if you look things up in other places, you need to know about this numbering problem.

The points in Table 11-1 help in alleviating pain in the upper/middle back, shoulders, and neck. In Table 11-2, you discover points for helping with low back pain and sciatica. Figure 11-1 shows the points for both tables.

When you look at Tables 11-1 and 11-2, you may wonder what those points are that are in parentheses. They're the numbers for the points used in the alternate numbering system. You can ignore them; we put them there in case you're also referencing other books while you learn acupressure.

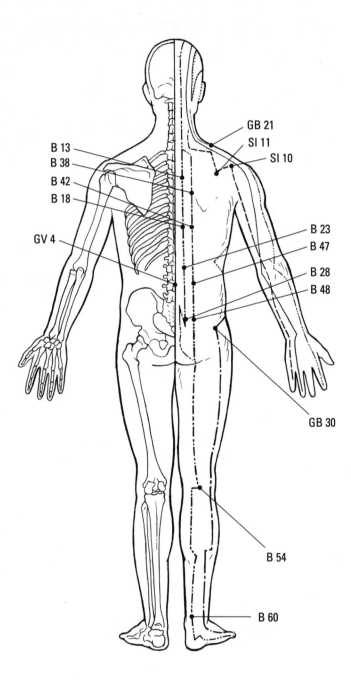

Figure 11-1:
The bladder
meridian
and corre-
sponding
acupoints.

You may want to take a few minutes before locating points to review your anatomy in Chapter 3. We use a lot of anatomical terms locating points along the back. Also, if you aren't sure what a chon is (or how to measure it), refer to Chapter 3.

Table 11-1		Upper and Mid Back Points	
Point Abbreviation	*Name of Point*	*How You Find It*	*Benefits*
B 13	Lu Shu	On the inside bladder line, one chon away from the spine, below the third thoracic vertebrae.	Relieves muscle spasms in the neck and upper back, reducing pain and discomfort.
B 38 (43)	Vitality Shu	On the outside bladder line, one and a half chon outside and one chon below B 13. It lies halfway between the top and bottom of the scapula, and halfway between the scapulae and the spine on the edge of the erector spinae muscle.	Relieves shoulder and upper back pain, and reduces tension and pain in the rhomboid muscles.
B 18	Liver Shu	On the inner bladder line, two chon below the inferior angle of the scapula, on the inside edge of the erector spinae muscle.	Excellent for relieving muscle spasms in the lower traps and erector spinae muscle group.
B 42 (47)	Spirit Door	On the outer bladder line, one and a half chon outside B 18.	Use for mid back pain, postural stress, and back stiffness.
SI 11	Celestial Gathering	In the middle of the shoulder blade.	Relieves shoulder tension.
SI 10	Outer Arm Bone	On the outside of the shoulder blade, below the point of the shoulder where the arm and shoulder come together.	Relieves headache, shoulder, and neck pain.

Table 11-2		Points for Easing Low Back Pain and Sciatica	
Point Abbreviation	Name of Point	How You Find It	Benefits
B 23	Kidney Shu	On the inner bladder line, in the middle of the waist, halfway between the rib cage and the hipbone, on the inner edge of the erector spinae muscle group.	Provides relief for low back pain, and reduces muscles tension.
B 47 (52)	Will's Chamber	On the outer bladder line, in the middle of the waist on the outside of the erector muscle group.	Provides relief for low back pain, and reduces muscle tension in the quadratus lumborum muscle.
B 28	Bladder Shu	On the inner bladder line, halfway between the top and bottom of the sacrum, and halfway between the inner and outer edge.	Used for buttock, sacral, and lower back pain. Relieves sciatica.
B 48 (54)	Bladder Vitals	On the outer bladder line, three chon to the side of the sacrum in the middle of the gluteal muscles of the buttocks. Very tender point.	Used for buttock, sacral, and lower back pain. Relieves sciatica.
B 54 (40)	Middle Crook	Right in the middle of the crease in the back of the knee.	Relieves low back pain, stiffness, and tension; used for sciatica and herniated discs; moves qi through the knee, reducing muscle spasms, knee pain, and stiffness.
GB 30	Jumping Round	Divide the sacrum in half from top to bottom. Find the edge of the sacrum with your thumbs, and slide three-quarters of the way into the gluteus muscles from the middle of the sacrum about one palm-width or four chon.	Reduces hip joint inflammation; relieves muscle sprains and pain; used for sciatica; reduces muscle spasms; relieves lower abdominal and lower back pain.

Point Abbre-viation	Name of Point	How You Find It	Benefits
B 60	Kunlun Mountains	Halfway between the Achilles tendon and the outer anklebone.	Relieves back pain and stiffness in the neck, the upper and lower back, and the leg.
GV 4	Life Gate	Between the vertebrae at the waistline at the same level as B 23.	Relieves lumbar back pain.

Acupressure routine to relieve back tension and pain

Here's a great routine to relieve stress and muscle tension along the whole back. At the end we add some specific points for sciatic pain and for assisting disk healing. Before starting, be sure that you have a sock filled with two tennis balls or your tools for reaching back points (see Chapter 2). Also, you'll be using the points in Table 11-2, which you can locate in Figure 11-1.

1. **Do your belly breathing while grounding and centering.**

2. **Do stretches for the bladder meridian and back.**

   Use your favorite back stretch or use either one of these stretches:

   - **Stand with your legs open to shoulder width.**

     Inhale and raise your arms over your head, gently leaning backward and stretching the front of your body.

     Exhale and bend forward, reaching your hands to the floor. Try to place your hands flat on the floor, raising your head to increase the stretch along your bladder meridian.

     Hang like a rag doll, breathing normally, and bouncing gently as you relax all the muscles in your back.

     Stretch to the right side, leaning over the right leg and holding the stretch for 20 seconds. Then walk your hands across the floor to your left leg and stretch over your left leg, holding it for 20 seconds.

- **Sit on the floor with your legs together, stretched out in front of you.**

  Lift your arms over your head while inhaling, and then exhale and bend forward, over your outstretched legs. Try to keep your back straight and lean out over your leg rather than folding your upper body. You can assist the stretch by grasping your toes with your hands. If you can't reach, use a towel; hold both ends and make a sling around your feet.

3. **Work all the points on both the inside and outside bladder lines.**

   You can work these points in several ways:

   - **Use your tennis ball sock tool while lying on your back by following these directions:**

     Lie on your back and place your tennis ball sock under your neck.

     Bend your legs so that your feet are flat on the floor. Gently raise your hips and back off the floor, so that you're balancing your weight on the tennis balls.

     Walk yourself up the tennis balls, so that they put pressure on your bladder points.

     Stop wherever you're sore and rock back and forth on the balls to work the tension out.

     When you finish the inside bladder line, untie the sock and re-tie it so that the tennis balls are more loosely held together. They should have enough room to separate and reach both outer bladder lines, just on the outside of the erector muscles on both sides of the spine.

   - **You can use your tennis ball sock tool while standing by following these directions:**

     Stand against a wall with your legs wider than shoulder width apart, knees bent at a 90 degree angle, as if you're sitting on an imaginary chair.

     Lean forward and place the tennis ball sock under your shoulders along the inside bladder line.

     Lean against the sock as you slowly straighten your legs, moving different parts of your back over the balls. As before, stop wherever you have soreness and roll up and down, massaging these points with the balls.

     Repeat for the outside bladder line.

- **You can also work these points while sitting in a chair with a tall back.**

  Start with the sock under your neck; roll around to relieve tension.

  Lean forward just a bit and let the balls fall down your back. Remember how close the bladder points are to each other, and don't let the balls fall more than an inch.

  Lean back and roll around on these new spots.

  Continue leaning forward and rolling until you've covered the whole back.

  Do the same with the outside bladder line.

- **You can use your back massage tool with the curved handle and the knobby end.**

  Place the knobby end on the bladder points and stimulate each individually. This method may take some time, so hang out only with the points that are really sore!

4. **Create even more relief by using the points in Tables 11-1 and 11-2 with the method of your choice — bilateral or one meridian at a time (check out Chapter 4 for more info).**

   You don't need to hold every point, just the ones that are calling you. And don't forget to try these on a friend too.

Reflexology for back stress and pain

The following reflexology routine can be effective in alleviating back pain and stiffness. You use the reflex areas included in Figure 11-2.

1. **Start by washing and drying your feet.**

2. **If you haven't already stretched and performed deep breathing exercises, do some deep belly breathing now.**

3. **Sit in a chair or on a bed and cross your leg so that you can hold your foot in your lap.**

4. **Warm, stretch, and open your feet by first rolling your foot back and forth in your hand, and then stripping your foot from top to bottom.**

   Repeat three or four times to reduce restrictions.

5. **Move your thumbs down to your heel and do thumb-walking along the reflex points for the entire spine and the sciatic nerve (see Figure 11-2).**

   The spine is the narrow strip on the inside of your foot running from your heel to your toe. The heel portion of the strip represents the small of your back; the middle part, in the arch of your foot, represents your waist; the upper part of the strip before your big toe represents your upper back. The base of the toes represents your neck. You find the sciatic nerve on the heel.

6. **If any spots are sore, use circular motions to work them out.**

7. **If any of the joints are inflamed, be sure to thumb-walk up the lymphatic strip along the outside of the foot, followed by circular motions on sore areas.**

8. **Repeat with the other foot.**

9. **Relax by lying quietly and feeling the flow of energy along your back. You may notice heat or tingling as qi flow balances.**

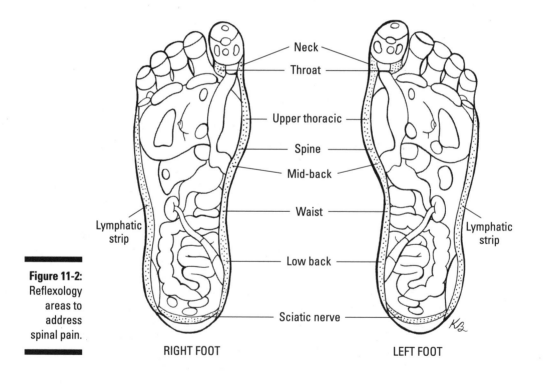

Figure 11-2:
Reflexology
areas to
address
spinal pain.

Chapter 12

Relief for Hurting Heads (And Pains in the Neck)

The area of your body above your shoulders occupies a relatively small portion of your total body, yet it's home to a considerable number of the chronic and painful conditions that plague people every day.

Maybe you have that headache that seems to strike almost every afternoon like clockwork, usually after a long and stressful day on the job. Or perhaps you have that dull pain in your jaw that strikes so often that you just take it for granted. Or maybe you've been plagued with earaches for as long as you can remember. For a relatively small area, the head and neck region has the potential to cause all sorts of painful problems that can really affect your quality of life in a negative way.

That's the bad news. The good news is that because so many of the problems in this area are related to excess muscle tension and vascular imbalance, they respond very well to acupressure and reflexology. Acupressure points in this area are easy to access and require very little pressure to impact. In fact, a lot of people rely on bodywork to provide the much-needed relief from these painful conditions that allows them to enjoy a relatively comfortable and happy life. In this chapter, we tell you about the most common problems associated with these parts of the body, and you learn techniques that can help you deal with the pain these problems can cause.

Going Whole Head: Treating the Entire Extremity

How do you deal with everyday tasks and responsibilities when your head and/or neck is killing you? Not very easily. And not with your usual care and attention, most likely. Pain in these areas is particularly disruptive because it can totally destroy your ability to concentrate and focus on the things you need to do. In addition, pain anywhere in your head or neck may affect your vision, hearing, and other senses that are necessary for you to absorb and process basic information, which is why we provide treatments for those specific areas later in this chapter. Bottom line: Head and neck pain can really wreak havoc on your life. So in this section, we take a closer look at the types of problems involved — and, more importantly, how you can deal with them.

Differentiating between types of headaches

People suffer from many different types of headaches, and those headaches have just as many different causes. The basic cause of a headache is generally the constriction of blood vessels and muscles (mainly in the head), which sends pain to the affected area. In some cases — especially with sinus headaches — the pain may be caused by an infection or injury. Of course, emotional stress, anxiety, depression, and other situational factors can also cause (or worsen) a headache.

✔ **Tension headache:** As the name implies, this type of headache often seems to be triggered by stress or frustration. The pain associated with a tension headache can vary from dull to severe, and is often described as a pressing or squeezing sensation. These headaches are usually caused by excess muscle tension in the neck, which presses on nerves, causing nerve pain, and presses on arteries, decreasing circulation into the head, which causes more pain. Acupressure and reflexology help by reducing muscle tension, taking pressure off nerve endings, and increasing circulation.

Tension headaches are extremely common. In fact, close to 80 percent of the population experiences a tension headache at some point in their life, according to the National Headache Foundation.

✓ **Migraine headache:** This is a severe headache that can often be debilitating, making it almost impossible to function normally. When suffering with a migraine headache, people may be nauseous or dizzy and experience severe pain on one or both sides of the head. Frequently, they're also very sensitive to noise and bright lights. Some evidence suggests that migraines may be hereditary. Migraine headaches are triggered by many things, including stress, hormone imbalance, pulsating light, foods, caffeine, alcohol, allergies, and more. The cause of these headaches is vascular — either too much or too little blood flow in the head — as opposed to tension. However, extreme muscle tension in the neck can disrupt blood flow to the head, contributing to the onset of a migraine. Many times, migraines are initiated by multiple triggers. Acupressure and reflexology help by balancing the circulation and reducing stress and muscle tension. The balancing effect of acupressure and reflexology on hormones may also be helpful.

According to the National Headache Foundation, one in four American households contains a migraine sufferer.

✓ **Sinus headache:** Sinus headaches are often brought on by a sinus infection, allergies, or related conditions. Not surprisingly, this type of headache involves pain close to the sinuses (nose, cheekbones, forehead) and can cause teeth pain, frontal headaches, and eye pain. Acupressure and reflexology can help in the longer term by supporting the immune system to fight the infection. In the short term, they help by reducing pain through the release of endorphins and by opening the sinuses to drain.

✓ **Cluster headache:** This type of headache gets its name from the fact that the headaches tend to come in groups. This is a very intense type of headache that often comes in a series (a person may experience several headaches within a day or two). It often involves excruciating pain behind or around one eye, possibly radiating to the temple on the same side, and may include a drooping eyelid. This headache is considered one of the worst types of pain and, like migraines, may include vomiting and sensitivity to light. Cluster headaches occur at the exact same time of the day on consecutive days or the same time and day, one week later. No one knows what causes them, but the regularity and timing suggest that they're related to a person's biological clock, or circadian rhythm. The circadian rhythm is a 24-hour cycle of changing physiologic processes that relate to sunlight and season.

Headaches may be common, but that doesn't mean they should be taken lightly, especially when they seem unusual for any reason. Some signs of trouble include dizziness, nausea, vision problems, and slurred speech. If you experience any of these symptoms with a headache — especially in the case of a very severe headache, or one that comes on suddenly — you should seek medical treatment right away. Likewise, you should consult a doctor about any headaches that follow a fall, head injury, or other trauma to the head or neck area.

Understanding the cause of neck pain

Go a little lower down the body, and you have the neck. It can be a great body part in many ways. It's a great showcase that conveniently displays the sparkling new necklace you love so much. And it's also the perfect spot for that beloved youngster in your life to wrap her arms around you for a goodnight hug.

Unfortunately, discomfort and soreness are also pretty common in this area. Sometimes you have pain due to something minor, perhaps even silly. Maybe you fell asleep while leaning over the side of your favorite recliner. Sure you may have slept like a baby, but a careless move like that can leave you paying the price (and rubbing your sore neck) for days.

Neck pain occurs for lots of different reasons, ranging from the small (sleeping funny) to the serious (arthritis, meningitis, and other unpleasant things). Injuries, accidents, and muscle strains are also common causes of neck pain.

If you experience neck pain, be sure to stay alert for any unusual signs of possible trouble. These signs could include any sudden loss of bladder or bowel function/control (which indicates neurological problems). Another red flag? A stiff neck that triggers pain when you drop your chin to your chest can sometimes indicate meningitis. If your neck pain is accompanied by numbness or shooting pain that extends down the arms or legs, it can also be a sign of serious problems that need to be addressed right away. If you experience any of these situations, see your doctor immediately.

Finding relief in the head and neck region: It's all in the yang points

All the points in the head and neck are yang points and tend to have excess energy. Yang meridians are the meridians that start in the head and face, traveling down the back of the body and backs of the arms. Almost all points above the collarbone in the front and above the shoulders in the back are on yang meridians. This means that they're likely to be active and full of qi. For a full discussion on the difference between yin and yang points, see Chapter 1.

In this section, we provide a routine to address all those nasty headaches we talk about in this chapter and the neck pain that often causes them. The different types of headaches have many common features, and their pain can be relieved by the following routine. Figures 12-1, 12-2, and 12-3 show you where these points reside, and Table 12-1 explains what each point does and how you find it.

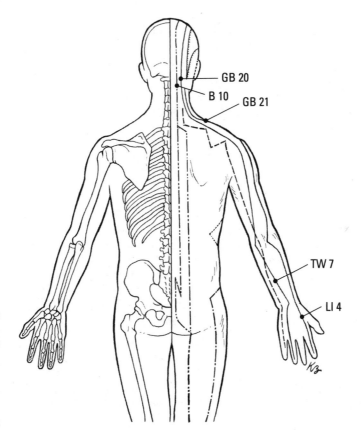

Figure 12-1:
Acupoints of
the arms,
hands, and
upper torso
(back).

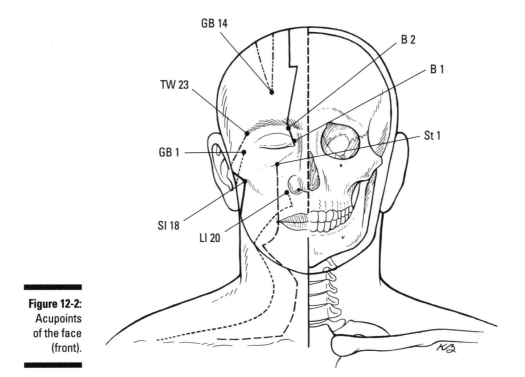

Figure 12-2:
Acupoints
of the face
(front).

Fibromyalgia can be a real pain in the neck

If you frequently experience pain in the neck (and possibly the shoulders, elbows, knees, and upper back) and can't seem to figure out what's causing it, perhaps you may be suffering from fibromyalgia.

Fibromyalgia is a syndrome in which the person (most commonly a woman) experiences diffused pain, fatigue, and a wide range of other symptoms, such as irritable bowel. The pain generally is most severe on 18 specific spots (commonly referred to as "tender points" because even the slightest touch can be painful), and then radiates out from that point into a more general region of the body.

A person must have pain in at least 11 of the tender spots to be diagnosed with fibromyalgia.

The pain of fibromyalgia often occurs in the shoulders and neck. It's not accompanied by any swelling or lumps, but you may have some stiffness in the affected areas. People with fibromyalgia often also have insomnia, fatigue, and other sleep-related problems.

The cause of fibromyalgia is unknown — and, unfortunately, it has no cure. However, many people find relief from their symptoms through bodywork, massage, chiropractic treatment, and over-the-counter or prescription pain relievers.

Controversy surrounds the diagnosis, treatment, and even existence of fibromyalgia. Until 20 years ago, the symptoms were thought to be all in the head of the sufferer. Even today many doctors don't recognize it as a legitimate condition, because it's diagnosed based on a set of symptoms that aren't related to a physiological cause. However, current research indicates that fibromyalgia may be a problem with the way the person's nerve cells transmit pain signals. Further research is needed to determine the cause of the syndrome before the medical community will fully recognize this debilitating chronic condition.

To learn more about fibromyalgia, see your doctor and check out *Fibromyalgia For Dummies,* by Roland Staud, MD, and Christine Adamec (Wiley).

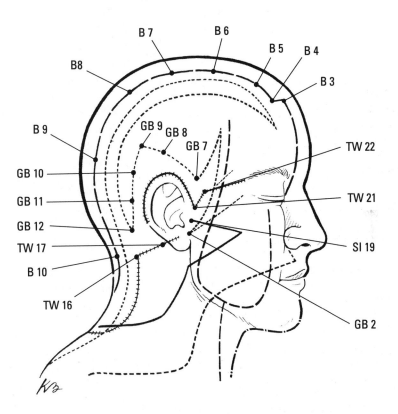

Figure 12-3:
Acupoints
of the face
(side).

Table 12-1		Acupoints to Release the Head and Neck	
Point Abbre-viation	**Name of Point**	**How You Find It**	**Benefits**
GB 21	Shoulder Well	In the top of the shoulder, halfway between the point of your shoulder and the base of your neck. In the belly of the muscle.	Relieves stiffness and pain in the neck, shoulder, and upper back.
GB 20	Wind Pool	Along the ridge of your occipital bone, halfway between your ear and spine; between the two muscles that come together (SCM and trapezius).	Subdues the liver meridian; use to reduce headache pain.
GB 12	Completion Bone	On the occipital ridge, in the depression behind the ear in the SCM muscle.	Use for head-aches, neck pain, and dizziness.
GB 6 GB 7 GB 8 GB 9 GB 10 GB 11	Suspended Tuft Hairline Curve Valley Lead Celestial Hub Floating White Head Portal Yin	A row of points that curl around the ear, starting at GB 12 and wrapping around to the top of the ear. The row is about one chon away from the ear. Hold all the points simul-taneously; you'll know when you reach them because they're sore.	Use for temporal headaches (on the side of your head) and migraines.
B 10	Heaven's Pillar	On the occipital ridge, just outside of where the spine enters the skull in the tendon.	Use for back-of-the-head head-aches, neck pain, and a stiff neck.
B 3 B 4 B 5 B 6 B 7 B 8 B 9	Eyebrow Ascension Deviating Turn Fifth Place Light Guard Celestial Connection Declining Connection Jade Pillow	A row of points on the head, one and a half chon to the side of midline. Start at B 10 and press and release all the points over the top of the head to the forehead.	Relieves occipital and frontal headaches and neck pain caused by arthritis.

Point Abbre-viation	Name of Point	How You Find It	Benefits
GB 14	Yang White	Go the middle of your eyebrow in line with the pupil of your eye when looking straight ahead. The point is one chon above the eyebrow.	Relieves frontal headaches and sinus headaches.
B 2	Bright Light	On the orbit of the eye on the inside of the eyebrow.	Excellent to relieve frontal and sinus headaches, and allergy symptoms.
LI 20	Welcome Fragrance	Just outside the nostril, pressing up into the cheekbone.	Opens sinuses and reduces sinus headaches and allergy symptoms.
TW 16	Celestial Window	In the muscle, under and slightly behind the earlobe.	Reduces neck stiffness and pain and relieves headaches.
LI 4*	Union Valley	This point is in the webbing between your thumb and index finger. It's traditionally located at the crease where your thumb and finger meet when you hold your fingers straight out and close your fingers and thumb together.	Reduces tension in the head and neck.

* Never use this point during pregnancy.

In the following routine, use the alternating pressure technique that we explain in Chapter 4 to disperse the energy in these points. If you don't have time for all the points, jump to the end of the routine, where we provide mini-sessions for specific types of headaches.

1. Belly breathe while centering and grounding (refer to Chapter 2).

2. Stretch out any overwork and tension by following these steps:

- Wrap a towel around your neck for support.

- Stretch by rolling in a full circle, three times in both directions.

- Stop anywhere it feels sore and hold the stretch for 20 seconds.

3. **Use the points in Table 12-1, starting with bilateral holds on GB 21, GB 20, and GB 12.**

4. **Fan your fingers and press all the GB points (6–11) that wrap around the ear together.**

   Press and release these points until they lose their soreness.

5. **Bilaterally hold B 10.**

6. **Fan your fingers and press the bladder points that go over the top of the head (B 3–9).**

   Hold as many at one time as you can, pressing and releasing these points until they lose their soreness. Keep moving along the line until you've pressed all the points. Repeat the entire line of bladder points at least three times.

7. **Bilaterally hold GB 14, B 2, LI 20, and TW 16.**

8. **Alternately hold LI 4 on each hand.**

9. **Use the following mini-healing sessions for specific headaches:**

   • **Tension Headache:** Use bilateral pressure on GB 21, GB 20, and GB 12; fan your fingers over GB 6–11 and then over B 3–9, working these points bilaterally. End holding LI 4 alternately on each hand. This mini-session reduces tension in the neck and head muscles that can cause tension headaches.

   • **Migraine Headache:** Bilaterally press B 10, TW 16, and GB 12. Fan your fingers over GB 6–11, compressing and releasing until sensitivity diminishes. Don't use too much pressure on these points or hold them for too long. End by pressing GB 14, followed by LI 4 on each hand. This helps balance blood flow into the head and regulates gall bladder qi. (If you're experiencing nausea with your migraine headache, HP 6 is a great anti-nausea point. Although we don't show it in this routine, you can find it in the routine in Chapter 6, and locate it in Figure 6-2.)

   • **Sinus Headache:** Use bilateral pressure on GB 20 and GB 17. Go back and forth on these points until they feel soft and have less soreness. Then press the following points bilaterally: SI 18, LI 20, St 1, B 1, B 2, and GB 14. End with LI 4 on each hand. This pattern helps relieve the pain of a sinus headache and opens the sinuses to drain.

   • **Cluster Headache:** The points that are sore in a cluster headache can be so tender that you don't want to touch them, so you can choose points above and below the pain to balance nerve and vascular function. On the side of your pain, hold GB 14 with GB 20; then hold B 2 with B 10. Fan your fingers over GB 6–11. End with LI 4 on both hands. If the pain is clustered around your eyes, check out Table 12-2 for help with eyestrain.

10. **Whatever session you do, end with 5 to 10 minutes of relaxation, or more if you have time.**

Relaxing allows the qi and blood flow to balance and stabilize before you become active again, and gives you time to appreciate those pain-relieving endorphins.

Relief for Eyestrain

Eyestrain can cause minor eye problems — such as blurred vision, pain in the muscles around the eyes, night blindness, and other conditions — that can be not only painful, but also very disruptive. Think about how much you rely on your eyes for virtually everything you do, throughout the entire day. Even a minor eye problem can really make your life much more challenging and frustrating than it needs to be.

Fortunately, simple strain and overexertion are often temporary and easily treated.

Eye problems that come on severely and suddenly should be monitored closely — especially if their onset coincides with other troublesome signs like slurred speech or a severe headache.

In the following routine, you use the points included in Table 12-2 and located in Figures 12-2 and 12-3, which we include earlier in the chapter.

Table 12-2		Points for Eye Relief	
Point Abbre-viation	**Name of Point**	**How You Find It**	**Benefits**
TW 16	Celestial Window	In the muscle, under and slightly behind the earlobe.	Reduces blurred vision, pain in the eyes, and tearing eyes.
TW 23	Silk Bamboo Hole	On the outside of the orbit of the eye, in the small notch felt toward the lateral eyebrow.	Helps all eye diseases, improves blurred vision, and reduces eye pain.
GB 1	Pupil Bone Hole	On the orbit of the eye at the corner of the outer eye.	Helps reduce light sensitivity and improves night blindness.
St 1	Tears Container	On the orbit of the eye, directly under your pupil when you're looking straight ahead.	Used for eye diseases, decreases eye twitching, and improves night blindness.

(continued)

Table 12-2 (continued)

Point Abbre-viation	Name of Point	How You Find It	Benefits
B 1	Bright Eyes	Inside corner of the eye in the bridge of the nose.	Reduces blurred vision, helps glaucoma and other eye disorders, and improves night blindness and vision problems.
B 2	Bright Light	On the orbit of the eye on the inside of the eyebrow.	Improves blurred vision, weak eyesight, excessive tearing, and general eye disorders.

Use this routine to alleviate the discomfort associated with eyestrain:

1. **Belly breathe while centering and grounding.**

2. **Look up, look down, look all around.**

   Exercise your eyes by looking as far as you can to the left, to the right, up, and then down. Do this slowly and really stretch your eye muscles. Afterward, slowly roll your eyes in a clockwise direction, and then in a counterclockwise direction.

3. **Locate the pressure points in Table 12-2 for clear vision:**

   • Use a bilateral hold on each point.

   • Spend as much time as you need to release each point.

   • When you're finished, rub your hands briskly together and place your palms over your eyes for 1 to 3 minutes.

   • Relax to allow the qi to balance and to let the tension drain from your eyes, fully receiving the benefits of the session.

Toning Down Tinnitus and Other Ear Problems

Ear problems are another fairly common source of pain and discomfort. Some typical causes of pain include the following:

✔ **Wax and fluid:** Fluid in the ear can be the source of uncomfortable pressure imbalances, especially when flying, or even traveling up a large hill.

A variety of over-the-counter treatments can help eliminate fluid and wax in the ear. Ear infections and more serious problems need to be treated by your doctor.

✔ **Tinnitus:** Tinnitus is a distracting and debilitating ringing or rushing sound in the ears. The cause of tinnitus is often unknown, although it can be a symptom of a more serious problem; acupressure and reflexology have been helpful in reducing the annoying sounds.

✔ **Loss of balance and vertigo:** Loss of balance can be due to fluid in the ear or disruption of normal fluid movement in the inner ear. Vertigo is a very debilitating condition where the room appears to be spinning, causing loss of balance, nausea, and disorientation.

Although medical treatment is usually necessary or helpful for ear problems, acupressure and reflexology techniques can prove to be a helpful addition in alleviating pain and noises in your ear(s).

If you experience ear pain accompanied by any type of discharge or bleeding from the ear, or any redness or swelling in the area around the ear, seek medical treatment right away.

In this section, you use the points included in Table 12-3, and illustrated in Figures 12-1 and 12-3, which we include earlier in this chapter.

Table 12-3		Acupoints to Hear By	
Point Abbreviation	*Name of Point*	*How You Find It*	*Benefits*
TW 7	Ancestral Gathering	On the back of the arm, one palm-width from the crease of the wrist on the outside of the tendon.	Use for deafness, tinnitus, and general ear disorders.
TW 16	Celestial Window	In the muscle, under and slightly behind the earlobe.	Use for swollen face, sudden deafness, and dizziness.
TW 17	Wind Screen	Directly under the earlobe on the skull bone, just before it meets the jawbone.	Use for deafness, tinnitus, earaches, and vertigo.

(continued)

Table 12-3 *(continued)*

Point Abbreviation	Name of Point	How You Find It	Benefits
TW 21	Ear Gate	In front of and at the top of the opening of the ear.	Use for deafness, tinnitus, ear disease, ear infections, and earaches.
TW 22	Harmony Bone-hole	Go to the bone one-half chon in front of the opening of the ear, and then up one chon in the muscle above the cheekbone.	Use for tinnitus and earaches.
SI 19	Hearing Palace	Directly in front of the opening of the ear, in the depression.	Use for ear disorders, deafness, tinnitus, ear infections, and vertigo.
GB 2	Hearing Meeting	Directly below SI 19.	Good for ear diseases, deafness, and tinnitus.

Try this routine to alleviate the discomfort of tinnitus and other ear problems:

1. **Belly breathe while centering and grounding.**

2. **Grasp both ears in your hands and gently but firmly rotate the ears.**

   Take a hold on the inside of the ear and gently pull the ear out. Walk your way all around the inside of the ear, gently pulling outward.

3. **Pressure points to hear by include the points in Table 12-3:**

   - Alternately hold TW 7 on both arms, maintaining pressure for up to 3 minutes.
   - Bilaterally hold TW 16, TW 17, TW 21, TW 22, SI 19, and GB 2.
   - Use alternating pressure on each point as long as it needs to release.
   - If you have a specific problem, refer to Table 12-3 and use the points that are specific to your need.
   - When you're finished, rub your hands briskly together and hold them over your ears for 1 to 3 minutes.
   - Relax by sitting or lying quietly while the qi you have stimulated balances the area.

Getting Cheeky and Chomping on Jaw Pain

Sure, you've probably heard the expression, "Put on a happy face." But trying to look happy can be nearly impossible when your face seems to be working against you. If you have pain in the facial area, a smile may seem like an impossible dream. Luckily, we have some techniques that may just help you turn that frown upside down.

In addition to your run-of-the-mill facial tension (think back to all those prom photos you had to smile endlessly for and the cheek exhaustion you may have felt afterward), many people experience jaw pain. TMJ is the abbreviation for the temporomandibular joint, commonly known as the jaw joint. You have a TMJ joint on each side of your face. It connects your jaw to your skull and allows your jaw the mobility it needs in order to talk, chew, and make pretty much any other kind of facial movement.

Although the term technically refers to the joint itself, TMJ is also the umbrella term commonly used to refer to several conditions involving the jaw and surrounding muscles and tissues. It can be tough to diagnose TMJ conditions, though, because pain in the jaw and facial region can be caused by many different things, including headaches, ear problems, dental problems, and others. In addition to pain in the jaw joint, a common symptom of TMJ conditions is a clicking or popping noise when opening and closing the mouth.

Doctors believe that stress can often be partially responsible for TMJ or for worsening its symptoms. For example, if a person tends to grind his jaw or clench his teeth when he's angry or stressed, it takes its toll on the jaw area and may trigger TMJ conditions.

Muscle tension can pull on the joints, stress can cause teeth grinding that wears on the joint, and arthritis in the joint can produce pain. Acupressure and reflexology have been very successful in reducing the symptoms of TMJ. Table 12-4 explains some helpful acupoints for treating facial pain; you can locate these points in Figures 12-2 and 12-3, earlier in this chapter.

Table 12-4		Acupoints for the Jaw and Face	
Point Abbre-viation	**Name of Point**	**How You Find It**	**Benefits**
TW 17	Wind Screen	Directly under the earlobe on the skull bone, just before it meets the jawbone.	Use for facial pain, lock jaw, trigeminal neuralgia, and nerve damage.
TW 21	Ear Gate	In front of the ear on the side of the face.	Good for TMJ and joint pain.
GB 1	Pupil Bone Hole	On the orbit of the eye at the corner of the outer eye.	Use for trigeminal neuralgia, facial paralysis, and Bell's palsy.
GB 2	Hearing Meeting	In front of the opening of the ear, just below TW 21.	Good for reducing effects of TMJ.
SI 18	Cheekbone Hole	At the lower edge of the cheekbone. Straight down from the outer corner of the eye and straight across from the lower edge of the nose.	Use for facial paralysis Bell's palsy, tooth-aches, and jaw swelling.

The following routine includes points that reduce muscle tension around the joint and disperse stagnant qi contributing to arthritis. All the points are stress reducing as well.

1. **Belly breathe while centering and grounding.**

2. **Exercise your face by following these steps:**

   • First, contract all the muscles in your face; scrunch up your mouth, your eyes, and your forehead. Squeeze all the muscles as tight at you can.

   • Then open everything as wide as you can; open your mouth, stretch your lips, widen your eyes.

3. **Follow these steps to get a good stretch:**

   • Relax and place your hands over the sides of your face, covering as much of your face as you can.

   • Pull your skin upward, and then downward; forward, and then backward. Hold each stretched position for 30 seconds to 1 minute.

4. **Bilaterally hold each of the points in Table 12-4.**

5. **Briskly rub your hands together and place them over your face for 1 to 3 minutes.**

6. **Relax to receive the greatest benefit while allowing qi flow to balance.**

Reflexology for the Head, Face, and Neck

Reflexology can be very helpful in alleviating many types of pain in the head, neck, and face. Here's an easy routine to try:

1. **Wash and dry your feet.**

2. **If you haven't already stretched and performed deep breathing exercises, do some deep belly breathing now.**

3. **Sit in a chair or on a bed and cross your leg so that you can hold your foot in your lap.**

4. **Use the reflex areas on the foot for the shoulders, neck, head, ears, eyes, lymphatic strip, and face (see Figure 12-4).**

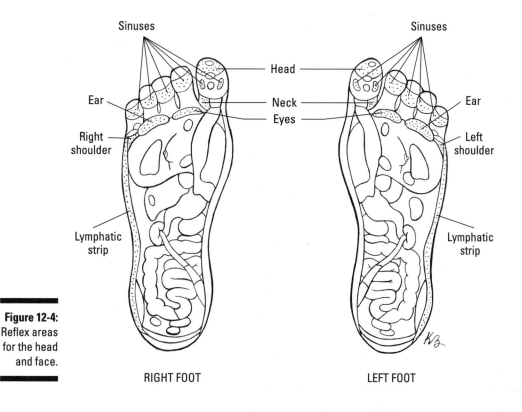

Figure 12-4:
Reflex areas
for the head
and face.

RIGHT FOOT   LEFT FOOT

5. **Press and massage the pads of your foot at the base of each toe, and then pull out to the end of the toes.**

6. **Thumb-walk and use circular motions all along the pads of the foot and toes to detect and release any imbalances.**

7. **Repeat with the other foot.**

8. **Relax by lying quietly and breathing deeply.**

   Let your body integrate the benefits of your healing session. As with all sessions, you may notice warmth spreading to the organs you stimulated.

Chapter 13

Lending a Hand (And Arm and Shoulder, Too!)

In This Chapter

▶ Zooming in on shoulder ailments

▶ Alleviating elbow problems

▶ Easing the pain of arthritis

▶ Helping hands and fingers

*Y*our arms and shoulders perform countless stressful tasks throughout the day — examples include typing on the computer, sewing, playing baseball, ironing, and more. Most people use their hands for things that involve repetitive motions, especially when they're on the job. Repetitive motions can be especially tough on the hands and fingers, and they can lead to specific painful conditions, such as carpal tunnel syndrome, while also aggravating existing conditions like arthritis.

Unfortunately, if you're like most people, you can't spend a few days refraining from using your arms or hands to give them a chance to recover from stress or injury. As a result, you further aggravate whatever problem caused the initial pain.

Discomfort in the hands and arms can make even the simplest daily tasks difficult and exhausting. Imagine trying to open a medicine bottle if your fingers are in serious pain. Or the sadness of being unable to lift your precious grandchild because your shoulder hurts too much.

Fortunately, we have some good news. By employing some acupressure and reflexology techniques, you can likely see considerable improvement in your arms and hands. And that opens up a whole new world of possibilities by allowing you to enjoy activities that may have been off-limits because they caused discomfort. If you're unsure of the root of your arm and hand pain, discuss it with your doctor, who may be able to determine the cause (and thus suggest some helpful treatment options).

Shouldering the Burden

Shoulder pain can have many different causes. The most common cause is muscle tension, often involving the *trapezius,* the muscle that pulls your shoulders to your ears when you're stressed out; the *rhomboids,* the muscles that pull the shoulder blade back; and the *pectoralis muscles,* which fight with the rhomboids to hunch the shoulders forward. (When that happens, your shoulders get caught in the middle!) Because the rhomboids are located on the back and the pectoralis muscles are on the chest, we provide routines for those aches in Chapters 11 and 15, respectively. The routine in this chapter effectively relieves the trapezius muscle, which most directly applies to your shoulder area.

Rotator cuff injuries and bursitis are two more conditions that can be improved with this routine. The *rotator cuff* muscles are a group of four muscles that rotate the shoulder, a ball and socket joint that can move in a full circle, through its range of motion. The more motion a joint has, the less stable it is, so these muscles work hard to provide both motion and stability. Common causes for rotator cuff injuries are overuse, repetitive use, and overextension. These are also the most common causes of bursitis, in which the *bursa* — the fluid-filled sacs inside the joint that protect the bones of the joint from rubbing against each other — become inflamed. The result? Excessive pain and discomfort and limited range of motion.

Don't let a frozen shoulder leave you out in the cold

Ever heard of a frozen shoulder? No, it's not what you get after a vicious snowball fight. Frozen shoulder is, in fact, a very serious and painful condition of the joint capsule causing pain and immobility of the shoulder. It's called *frozen shoulder* because it consists of limited range of motion in the joint. Usually the person can't lift the arm even to shoulder level in any direction. The exact cause is unknown; it can happen from an injury, overextending the arm, sitting down too hard in a chair, and so on. Sometimes it's the result of the area being immobilized for an extended period, such as after an accident or injury. It generally afflicts only one shoulder, and is more common among people who are middle-aged or older, and more common among women than men.

A frozen shoulder usually resolves in time; on average, it takes about six months. Physical therapy exercises to help release adhesions, lubricate the joint capsule, and strengthen surrounding muscles are very helpful. People with frozen shoulder often find relief with acupressure. Nourishing qi helps lubricate the joint and release muscle tension. Pain is often reduced and mobility increased after an acupressure session. The shoulders can also be worked with reflex areas on the feet or hand to stimulate the healing process.

The acupressure and reflexology routines in this chapter alleviate muscle tension and can speed the recovery time of these injuries. They increase circulation to the area and stimulate the body's healing processes. Increased circulation brings all the ingredients the body needs to heal and takes away the products of inflammation that get in the way of tissue repair.

You can use the healing techniques of acupressure to assist (and possibly prevent) some common shoulder problems. Use the points included in Table 13-1 and illustrated in Figure 13-1.

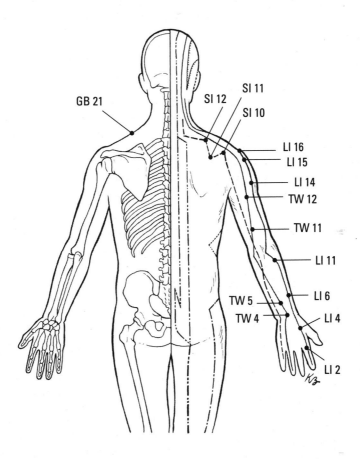

Figure 13-1:
Shoulder points in the arms, hands, and upper torso (back).

Table 13-1   Acupressure Points for Shoulder Stress and Bursitis

Point Abbreviation	Name of Point	How You Find It	Benefit
GB 21	Shoulder Well	In the top of your shoulder, halfway between the point of your shoulder and the base of your neck. In the belly of the muscle.	Relieves stiffness and pain in the shoulder and upper back.
LI 16	Giant Bone	At the joint where your collarbone meets your shoulder bone, on the neck side of the acromial joint.	Use for shoulder pain, bursitis, and rotator cuff injuries.
LI 15	Shoulder Bone	Directly on the point of your shoulder. When you raise your arm sideways, a dimple forms at the point. One chon on the arm side from LI 16.	Helps afflictions of the shoulder joint and muscles.
LI 14	Upper Arm Point	On the side of your arm, one palm-width from the point of your shoulder, in the deltoid muscle.	Relieves muscle aches and tension in the shoulder and arm.
SI 10	Outer Arm Bone	On the outside of your shoulder blade, below the joining of your arm and shoulder (at the armpit).	Improves pain, stiffness, and weakness in the shoulder blade, shoulder, and arm.
SI 11	Celestial Gathering	In the middle of your shoulder blade, halfway between the top and bottom, halfway between the inside and outside edges.	Use for pain and stiffness in the shoulder blade.
SI 12	Grasp the Wind	On the top of your shoulder blade, just above the bony ridge (spine of the scapula) and in the middle of the muscle, halfway between your neck and shoulder.	Use for all shoulder and shoulder blade disorders, including stiffness, pain, and numbness.

The following acupressure routine helps relieve stress, tension, and pain in the shoulders:

1. **Belly breathe while centering and grounding (refer to Chapter 2).**

2. **Stretch the meridians in the front and sides of the arms by following these steps:**

   • Stand with your feet shoulder-width — or farther — apart.

   • Bend your knees slightly.

   • Breathe in while raising your arms to shoulder level, with your palms down. Continue breathing in while spreading your arms backward at shoulder blade level and rotating your hands to a palms-up position. Reach your thumbs toward the floor behind you without bending backward.

   • Exhale and relax, bringing your arms back to your sides.

   • Repeat three times.

3. **Stretch the meridians in the back of the arm and shoulder meridians by following these steps:**

   • Clasp your hands together and raise them in front of you at shoulder height.

   • Swing side to side in time with your breathing, stretching your arms as you swing.

4. **Select the shoulder that needs the most care, and then use your opposite hand to press the points on the shoulder in the following sequences:**

   • GB 21, LI 16, LI 15, and LI 14.

   • SI 12, SI 11, and SI 10.

   • Use sustained pressure on points that feel empty, and use alternating pressure on points that feel full. Repeat each sequence several times until the points feel less painful.

5. **Repeat Step 4 with the other shoulder.**

6. **You can continue the session with points for the elbows and hands, or relax and enjoy the free flow of energy through your shoulders.**

Tennis Elbow, Anyone?

If you're an athlete or if you work with your arms and hands, you're a candidate for elbow problems. Roofers, carpenters, road workers, tennis players, lacrosse players, and even baseball players are subject to this problem. Repetitive use of the elbow contributes to both tennis elbow and golfer's elbow.

The funny bone: No laughing matter

It may have a humorous-sounding name, but to anyone who's ever suffered an injury to the area, the funny bone is anything but comical. The funny bone (or *olecranon,* as it's officially called) is an area of your elbow that seems to be particularly vulnerable to bumps and other injuries. It can also be the site of a painful condition called *olecranon bursitis,* which causes symptoms like tingling, pain, and swelling in the elbow region.

Tennis elbow is the common name for *lateral epicondylitis.* This condition affects the tendons on the outside of the elbow. It's the most common injury that results in elbow pain. Although nobody knows exactly what causes it, you're most likely to get it through repetitive use of your elbow.

If you're a golfer, you may be familiar with another, less frequent elbow strain: golfer's elbow. Golfer's elbow is the common name for *medial epicondylitis* and affects the tendons of the inside of the elbow. It's also caused by repetitive use.

Acupressure can help bring circulation and healing qi to elbow issues. We list acupressure points for the elbow in Table 13-2 and show them in Figures 13-1 and 13-2. If you're unfamiliar with using a chon as a measurement, check out Chapter 3 for details.

Table 13-2		Acupressure Points for the Elbow	
Point Abbreviation	*Name of Point*	*How You Find It*	*Benefits*
LI 11	Crooked Pond	At the top of the elbow crease, on the edge of the joint.	Relieves elbow pain, arthritis, and inflammation.
LI 4*	Union Valley	In the webbing where the index finger and the thumb meet. If you close your finger and thumb, you'll find it at the bottom of the crease. You can pinch this point between your index finger and thumb.	Alleviates pain and disperses excess tension.
H 3	Lesser Sea	On the inside (baby finger side) crease of your elbow at the tender spot.	Especially useful for pain involving the ulnar nerve, involved in golfer's elbow.

Point Abbreviation	Name of Point	How You Find It	Benefits
H 4	Spirit Path	On the palm side of the arm, one and a half chon above the crease of the wrist in line with the little finger.	Use for arm pain and muscle spasms.
TW 11	Clear Cold Abyss	On the back of the arm in the tendon of the triceps muscle, two chon (three finger-widths) up from the point of the elbow.	Use for pain in the shoulder, arm, and shoulder blade.
TW 12	Dispersing Brilliance	Halfway between the elbow and the shoulder in the triceps muscle.	Alleviates pain in the arm.

* Never use this point during pregnancy.

Here's a routine that can help address elbow problems. If you're adding the elbow points on to the shoulder-freeing routine from the earlier "Shouldering the Burden" section, start right in. If you're skipping the shoulder-freeing routine points, go back and do Steps 1, 2, and 3 in that routine before starting the elbow tendon points in this routine.

1. **Start with the elbow that needs the most attention, and use your opposite hand to give alternate pressure on the following pairs of points.**

   Work each pair until it feels less tense and then move on to the next pair.

   - LI 11 and LI 4
   - H 3 and H 4
   - TW 11 and TW 12

   Use sustained pressure on points that feel empty, or alternating pressure on points that feel full.

2. **Repeat with the other elbow.**

   Even if you don't have problems with the other elbow, doing the opposite side is always a good idea. This helps the body further relax and send qi to the side in need.

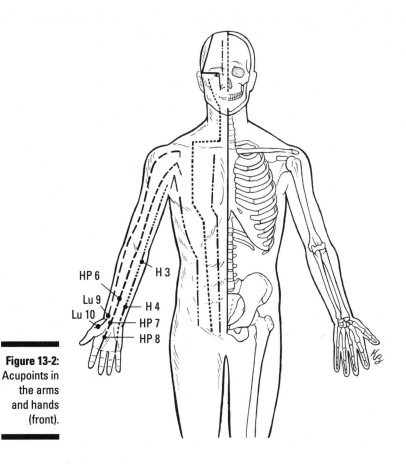

Figure 13-2:
Acupoints in
the arms
and hands
(front).

Help for Your Wrists and Hands

All too often the hands are the site of discomfort and pain from joint-degenerating conditions, such as osteoarthritis and rheumatoid arthritis. When you bring circulation and qi into the area, you can reduce stiffness, inflammation, and pain.

You can also try the ice treatment in Chapter 4, but only when your joints are hot and inflamed. Be careful not to overuse ice. In traditional Chinese medicine, too much cold can cause harmful side effects like stagnant qi, contributing to arthritis and other conditions that you may be trying to alleviate. You're using too much ice if you rely on it every time you feel pain. Using ice correctly means using it only when you have a hot, inflamed, painful joint or injury.

Maybe you're one of the many people who suffer from carpal tunnel syndrome. If so, the routine in this section may provide some relief.

Opening the tunnel in your carpal (and other wrist and hand issues)

Carpal tunnel can be a very painful condition. The *carpal tunnel* is a tunnel through your wrist in which tendons, arteries, veins, and nerves travel to get to the hands. The syndrome has many causes. The tunnel may collapse, in which case you may need surgical correction or physical therapy. Another cause of carpal tunnel syndrome is inflammation of the tendons going into the hand. This happens from overuse, especially with activities like computer work or video games. When the tendons inflame, they compress the median nerve going into your hand.

You may be surprised to learn that a popular pastime is being blamed for more and more cases of carpal tunnel. What is it? Video games. Doctors are reporting an increasing number of cases among kids and teenagers (groups rarely afflicted by this condition in previous times). Experts attribute this to the number of hours many kids today spend playing video games involving repeated finger movements to operate the controls.

The following routine for pain relief in the hands can be added to the shoulder and/or elbow routines. You can find points in Table 13-3 and in Figures 13-1 and 13-2. If you're not sure how to measure a chon, check Chapter 3.

Table 13-3	Acupoints for the Wrists and Hands		
Point Abbreviation	*Name of Point*	*How You Find It*	*Benefits*
LI 4*	Union Valley	In the webbing where the index finger and the thumb meet. If you close your finger and thumb, you find it at the bottom of the crease. You can pinch this point between your index finger and thumb.	Use to relieve pain and inflammation.

(continued)

Table 13-3 *(continued)*

Point Abbreviation	Name of Point	How You Find It	Benefits
LI 6	Deviated Passage	With your elbow bent at your side, rotate your arm so that the thumb is in the thumbs up position. The point is on the top surface (side) of your arm, three chon (one palmwidth) from your wrist in line with your thumb.	Relieves aching in the hand and arm.
TW 4	Yang Pool	Go to the back of the hand to the wrist and find the point in the middle of the crease halfway between the inside and outside of the wrist.	Use for pain in the arm, shoulder, and wrist.
TW 5	Outer Gate	Two chon (three finger-widths) above the wrist crease on the outside of the hand.	Use for pain when moving the shoulder, elbow, wrist, or fingers.
HP 6	Inner Gate	On the palm side of the hand, in the middle of the arm, two chon (three finger-widths) above the wrist crease.	Can be used for pain in the elbow, arm, and hand along the median nerve.
HP 7	Great Mound	Go to the palm side of the wrist and find the point halfway between the inside and outside of the wrist crease.	Benefits the wrist and median nerve.
HP 8	Labor Palace	In the middle of the palm of the hand, where your middle finger hits when you curl your hand.	Decreases heat sensations in the palm of the hand.

*Never use this point during pregnancy.

Try this acupressure routine to help alleviate some of the discomfort. If you're adding the carpal tunnel points to the shoulder-freeing routine from the earlier "Shouldering the Burden" section, start the following sequence. If you skipped the shoulder routine points, go back and do Steps 1, 2, and 3 from that routine before starting this one.

1. **Work the hand that needs the most attention first, and, using your opposite hand, alternately press the following point pairs, using alternating or sustained pressure as needed.**

   Work with each pair until it feels clear and then move to the next pair:

   - LI 4 and LI 6

   - TW 4 and TW 5

   - HP 6 and HP 7

2. **Hold TW 4 and HP 7 at the same time with sustained pressure for 3 minutes.**

3. **Hold TW 5 and HP 6 at the same time for 3 minutes.**

4. **End by holding HP 8 for 3 minutes.**

5. **Relax and enjoy the free flow of qi.**

Silencing the click of a trigger finger

Trigger fingers (or trigger thumbs) are identified by a characteristic clicking when you bend or straighten your finger or thumb. It occurs most often in the index finger and thumb. If you have a trigger finger, you know that in addition to clicking, it can lock in either a fully straightened or bent position.

Do you garden, play the piano, knit, or do detailed work with your hands? If so, you can be susceptible to trigger finger because it can be caused by repetitive use (again!). The tendons swell as they pass through the tendon sheath — a condition called *tenosynovitis*. If you have trigger finger, you may feel pain in your wrist as well as over the top of your finger.

In this section, we give you a routine that may help your trigger finger. The points you need are in Table 13-4, and you can locate them in Figures 13-1 and 13-2.

Table 13-4	Acupoints to Unlatch the Catch		
Point Abbreviation	**Name of Point**	**How You Find It**	**Benefits**
LI 2	Second Interval	On the outside of the index finger on the joint where the finger meets the hand, slightly toward the fingertip.	Use to reduce pain in index finger.
LI 4*	Union Valley	In the webbing where the index finger and the thumb meet. If you close your finger and thumb, you find it at the bottom of the crease. You can pinch this point between your index finger and thumb.	Disperses heat and releases tension in the thumb.
Lu 10	Fish Border	On the palm surface of the hand, halfway between the outside of the wrist and the first joint of the thumb in the fleshy part of the pad. It will be very tender.	Impacts the radial nerve and releases the muscles in the thumb pad.
Lu 9	Great Abyss	On the palm side of the hand, under the thumb, in the wrist crease.	Use to relieve pain in the wrist joint and fingers.
HP 8	Labor Palace	In the middle of the palm of the hand, where your middle finger hits when you curl your hand.	Decreases heat sensations in the palm of the hand.

* Never use this point during pregnancy.

Tormented by trigger finger? Here's a routine that may help. If you're adding the trigger finger points to the shoulder-freeing routine from the earlier "Shouldering the Burden" section, start the following sequence. If you skipped the shoulder routine points, go back and do Steps 1, 2, and 3 of that routine before starting the trigger finger routine. If you have time, doing these points after the carpal tunnel routine in the last section can be very beneficial.

1. **Start with the hand that needs the most attention, and, using your opposite hand, put alternate pressure on the following point pairs:**

   • LI 2 and LI 4

   • Lu 9 and Lu 10

2. **Use alternating or sustained pressure and continue to work with these two point pairs until they feel better.**

3. **End by holding HP 8 for 3 minutes.**

4. **Relax and experience the reduced tension in your muscles and tendons; you may want to gently stretch your trigger finger or thumb as the qi flow balances.**

Reflexology to the Rescue for Shoulders, Elbows, and Hands

Reflexology can be a great way to relieve tension and soreness in your shoulders, arms, and hands. As with all reflexology routines, you can use the reflex areas on either your feet or your hands. You may notice that there is no reflex area for the arms and hands; working the shoulders stimulates qi flow along the whole limb. You may prefer to do this routine on your hands because they're directly involved with the treatment. But be careful — don't aggravate your own sore hands by using them! You may want to get someone else to do it for you! You can benefit by using reflexology alone or by using it following the acupressure treatments in this chapter.

1. **Start by washing and drying your feet.**

2. **If you haven't already stretched and performed deep breathing exercises, do some deep belly breathing now.**

3. **Sit in a chair or on a bed and cross your leg so that you can hold your foot in your lap.**

4. **Roll your foot back and forth in your hand, loosening up any restrictions. Use horizontal stripping (see Chapter 4) to further open the zones of your foot.**

5. **Find the reflex zones for the shoulders, arms, and hands (see Figure 13-3).**

   You can find them under the baby toe on both feet.

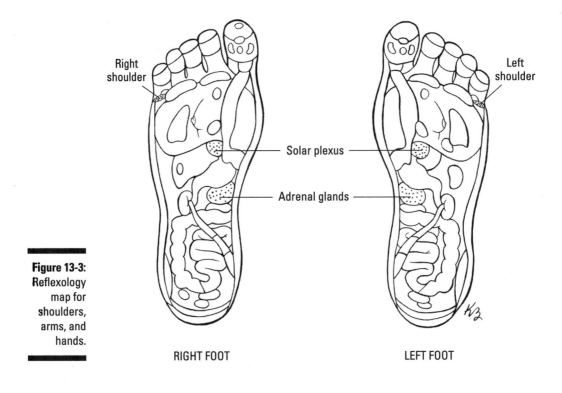

Figure 13-3: Reflexology map for shoulders, arms, and hands.

RIGHT FOOT   LEFT FOOT

6. **Thumb-walk the area looking for any nodules, soreness, or crackling sounds, and use circular motions to work out the tension.**

7. **End with thumb-walking and circular motions to the solar plexus and the adrenals to stimulate smooth qi flow.**

8. **Repeat with the other foot.**

9. **Lie still and let yourself feel the benefits of moving qi.**

   You may notice tingling, warmth, or relaxation. The longer you give yourself to integrate the session, the better your result will be.

Chapter 14

Time for a Gut Check

Most people use the generic term *stomachache* to refer to any type of abdominal pain or problem. But a wide variety of conditions can cause discomfort in this area. Many people suffer from one or more of a group of symptoms that could fall under the category of *digestive problems* and generally aren't the type of things people are eager to discuss: nausea, gas, constipation, and so on.

Digestive problems can result from many causes — a poor diet, obviously, is one. Even if your overall diet is generally good, you may have a sensitivity to a specific food or type of food. For example, many people have trouble digesting dairy products, while others have stomachs that aren't exactly thrilled with hot and spicy meals. Stress can also frequently disrupt the normal flow of your digestive process. An additional cause of digestive problems is invasion of microscopic pests such as bacteria. Of course, chronic medical conditions such as Irritable Bowel Syndrome (IBS) can also contribute to abdominal pain and digestive problems.

Determining the root cause of your digestive problems is difficult if all you have to go by are symptoms. Many causes produce the same symptom, so see your doctor for a diagnosis.

The ideal solution for stomach problems is to get your dietary routine in better shape — and that should definitely be your long-term goal. But in the meantime, bodywork techniques can help you cope with some of your stomach woes. This chapter tells you how.

How Bodywork Techniques Can Ease Symptoms of Poor Digestion

You're probably familiar with the symptoms of digestive problems. We're talking about all those nasty maladies the narrator rattles off during the typical commercial for an antacid or other stomachache remedy. Heartburn, sour stomach, indigestion, constipation, diarrhea, and other assorted intestinal problems all fall into this category.

For better or worse, these conditions tend to be blatantly obvious. In other words, if you're having trouble in the stomach area, you're probably painfully aware of it — usually immediately after the problem begins. The good news is that this awareness means you can also start treating the symptoms immediately, increasing your chances of rectifying the problem before it gets any worse.

Stomach ailments can be the result of excess stimulation to the digestive tract, or stimulation at times when it isn't needed. The cause? You guessed it — stress! Acupressure and reflexology are great at reducing stress, and they also help restore normal digestive function by restoring balance. Most important, acupressure helps the body do what it's already trying to do — heal itself — so you don't have to be an expert in knowing the cause of the problem. Use the routines in this chapter for any digestive upset to help restore balance.

Even some of the more severe digestive ailments, like Crohn's disease and colitis, can be improved with acupressure and reflexology. Most digestive disorders disrupt the lining of the digestive tract and create inflammation, decreasing the digestion and absorption of nutrients. Acupressure and reflexology can help the body's efforts to repair the digestive lining and reduce inflammation by increasing circulation and restoring harmonious qi flow.

Settling Digestive Disturbances with Acupressure

In Chinese medicine, disorders are treated by balancing the qi in unbalanced areas. The acupressure approach can work well in alleviating digestion-related discomfort.

Focus on the points in Figures 14-1, 14-2, and 14-3 — and read about them in Table 14-1 — for the acupressure routine in this section, which helps address digestion problems.

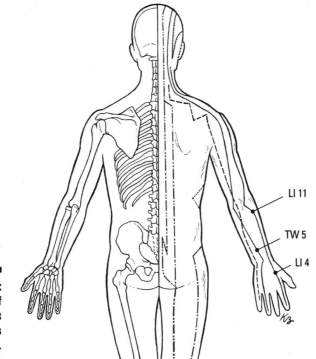

Figure 14-1:
Acupoints of
the arms
and hands
(back).

LI 11

TW 5

LI 4

Table 14-1		Points to Digestive Health	
Point Abbreviation	*Name of Point*	*How You Find It*	*Benefits*
LI 4*	Union Valley	In the webbing where the index finger and the thumb meet. If you close your finger and thumb, you find it at the bottom of the crease. You can pinch this point between your index finger and thumb.	Good for improving overall intestinal function, including diarrhea, constipation, and abdominal pain.

(continued)

Table 14-1 *(continued)*

Point Abbreviation	Name of Point	How You Find It	Benefits
LI 11	Crooked Pond	At the top of the elbow crease, on the edge of the joint.	Use for diarrhea, constipation, and abdominal pain.
TW 5	Outer Gate	Two chon (three finger-widths) above the wrist crease on the outside of the hand.	Helps relieve nausea, vomiting, and urinary incontinence.
HP 6	Inner Gate	Palm side of the hand, two chon (three finger-widths) above the wrist crease in the middle of the arm.	Improves stomachache, indigestion, nausea, vomiting, and anxiety.
St 36	Three Mile Point	One chon out from the shinbone and three chon below the patella.	This is an overall gastrointestinal tonic: It helps heal ulcers and relieves indigestion, enteritis, nausea, diarrhea, constipation, gas, and bloating.
Sp 4	Grandfather-Grandson	This point is on the side of the inside of the foot, one chon behind the base of the big toe. Find the bone in the arch of the foot, hook your finger into the arch from underneath, and press upward.	Harmonizes stomach qi; one of the best points to relieve indigestion, ulcers, stomachaches, and nausea.
Sp 6*	Three Yin Crossing	Three finger-widths above the inner anklebone, along the back of the tibia.	Helps all diseases of the lower abdomen: Used for ulcers, colitis, and all problems of the stomach and spleen. Relieves abdominal distention, diarrhea, constipation, and flatulence.

Point Abbreviation	Name of Point	How You Find It	Benefits
Lv 3	Great Rushing	On the top side of the foot, go between the big and second toes; trace up the webbing between the metatarsal bones until the bones come together forming a depression.	Relieves nausea, vomiting, abdominal pain, and distention. Improves gall bladder health.
CV 12	Middle Cavity	In the midline of the front of the body, halfway between the breastbone and belly button.	Helps all abdominal issues and is often used for indigestion, heartburn, abdominal pain, and constipation.

* Never use this point during pregnancy.

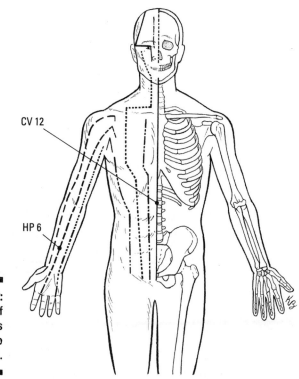

CV 12

HP 6

Figure 14-2:
Acupoints of
the arms
and torso
(front).

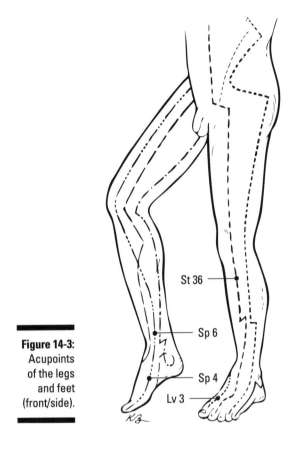

Figure 14-3:
Acupoints
of the legs
and feet
(front/side).

The following acupressure routine is effective for opening up the digestive channels and making your abdominal area more comfortable. Any digestive condition can benefit from the following routine. You can also focus the session by using only points whose functions are specific to your concern.

1. **Belly breathe while centering and grounding (refer to Chapter 2).**

2. **Stretch your whole body to open all the digestive channels.**

   • Take your arms up over your head while breathing in and stretch backward as far as it's comfortable (don't overstretch and hurt yourself!). Hold for the count of three.

   • Exhale as you bend forward, stretching your arms to the floor. Be a rag doll and hold this for the count of three.

- Inhale as you stand back up; bring your arms over your head and lean to the side, exhaling while you lean. Hold.

- Breathe in as you straighten up and repeat on the other side.

- Repeat the whole sequence three times to fully open all meridian channels.

3. **For overall digestive health, use all the points in Table 14-1 as follows:**

- Use the *one meridian at a time technique* (see Chapter 4) and hold LI 4, LI 11, TW 5, and HP 6. Hold each with alternating or sustained pressure for 1 to 3 minutes each, or until they feel open and without tension.

- Repeat these points on the other side of the body.

- Use the bilateral technique to hold St 36, Sp 4, Sp 6, and Lv 3. Hold each with alternating or sustained pressure for 1 to 3 minutes each, or until they feel open and without tension.

- Repeat any points that need additional attention.

- End by holding CV 12 for 1 to 3 minutes.

4. **If you don't have time for a full treatment or to address a specific intention, hold the following points with either a bilateral approach or one meridian at a time, whichever is easiest for you:**

- **Short overall treatment:** St 36, Sp 4, LI 11, LI 4

- **Nausea:** St 36, Lv 3, HP 6, TW 5

- **Diarrhea:** Sp 4, Sp 6, St 36, LI 4, LI 11

- **Constipation:** LI 11, LI 4, St 36, Lv 3, CV 12

- **Bloating:** Lv 3, Sp 6

- **Urinary incontinence:** TW 5

- **Indigestion:** CV 12, Sp 4, St 36

- **Ulcers:** St 36, Sp 4, Sp 6

5. **Rest and relax, or include a reflexology session.**

Resting after a session allows the qi to fully balance and restore harmony. The longer you rest and relax, the more effective the session will be.

Reflexology for Healthy Digestion

Reflexology is a great way to improve digestive symptoms. All the digestive organs can be stimulated through the hands and feet, encouraging better balance and overall function. In addition, reflexology acts through the nervous system. The nervous system and endocrine system are the master controllers of the digestive process, and this routine can help regulate nervous system control over digestive function. Use Figure 14-4 to find the reflex points for the digestive organs to use in this routine.

1. **Start by washing and drying your feet.**

2. **If you haven't already stretched and performed deep breathing exercises, do some deep belly breathing now.**

3. **Sit in a chair or on a bed and cross your leg so that you can hold your foot in your lap.**

4. **Roll your foot back and forth in your hand, loosening up any restrictions. Use horizontal stripping to further open the zones of your foot.**

5. **Find the reflex zones for all the digestive organs: the stomach, spleen, large intestine, small intestine, liver, gall bladder, and pancreas.**

   They're all located mostly in the arch of the foot.

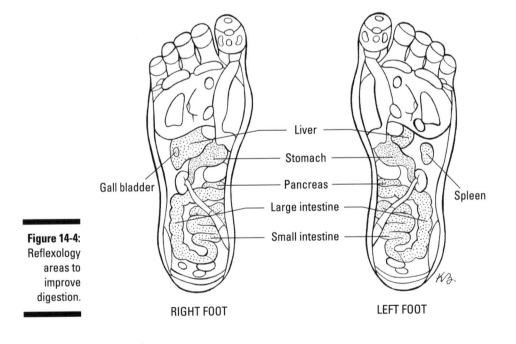

Figure 14-4:
Reflexology areas to improve digestion.

Gall bladder

Liver

Stomach

Pancreas

Large intestine

Small intestine

Spleen

RIGHT FOOT   LEFT FOOT

6. **Thumb-walk the organs looking for any nodules, soreness, or crackling sounds.**

7. **Use circular motions on any sore or nodular areas.**

8. **Repeat with the other foot.**

9. **Relax and allow your body time to respond to the changes you have started.**

   You may hear gurgles and other noises coming from your digestive tract. This is a great sign and means normal movement and function are being stimulated.

Chapter 15

Chest-Related Care and Considerations

....

In This Chapter

▶ Brushing up on breathing basics

▶ Breathing easier for better comfort

▶ Encouraging better respiratory function

▶ Knowing the essentials of heart health

....

*Y*ou could say that the chest is, literally and figuratively, the heart and soul of the body. First and foremost, it's where your heart hangs out and runs the entire operation. We don't think we need to explain why your heart is important — we're pretty sure that you're well aware of your heart's role in the grand scheme of things.

The chest is also home to the lungs, which provide the oxygen that makes all things possible, biologically speaking. Sure, you know that breathing is an important thing. If a person doesn't breathe, he quickly dies. But it's not as cut-and-dried as that. It isn't enough just to breathe; for optimal performance and vitality, you must breathe well. If your breathing is compromised in any way, it affects many of your other bodily functions. Your heart may need to work harder, your brain may struggle to perform without its necessary supply of fresh oxygen, and countless other anatomical processes may also be affected.

In this chapter, we tell you about some common causes of heart and lung problems. We tell you how acupressure and reflexology can help with these common problems, and we give you specific routines to help you get your heart and lungs into the best shape possible.

What Causes Heart and Lung Problems (And How Bodywork Can Help)

A variety of health conditions can cause (or worsen) heart and lung problems. High blood pressure, asthma, genetic conditions — these can all spell trouble for the heart and lungs, as can temporary/recurring problems such as bronchitis and pneumonia.

From a traditional Chinese viewpoint, many of these problems can also be caused by energy blockages or imbalances. Improper energy flow can, for example, cause poor circulation, which in turn causes the heart to work less efficiently and forces the lungs to work harder.

By restoring the proper flow of energy — and focusing on specific points that correspond with heart and lung function — you can greatly improve the way your body feels and performs.

Bodywork isn't intended to treat heart attacks or other critical emergencies. Should you experience any sudden chest pains, rise in blood pressure, or other symptoms of heart problems, seek medical treatment immediately.

When the blood pump gets weak

Many of the same things that pose a danger to your lungs (see the next section) can also threaten the health of your heart — things like smoking and pollutants. However, your heart faces additional dangers. For one thing, it's much more vulnerable to diet-related factors, such as too much cholesterol, fat, and sugar.

Diseases like diabetes, high blood pressure, hardening of the arteries (atherosclerosis), and kidney problems all put added strain on your heart. So too does the swelling in your feet that happens with varicose veins and other circulatory problems, causing the heart to work extra hard to move the fluid. On top of that, some people are born with congenital heart diseases or may develop defects such as faulty heart valves and arrhythmias that may need to be treated and monitored throughout their entire lives.

Ultimately, a healthy heart reflects healthy choices; lifestyle changes are key in correcting or managing heart problems. Acupressure and reflexology are great tools to support you and your heart in this effort — they contribute to heart health in the following ways:

✔ **They decrease blood pressure.** These techniques promote relaxation of the smooth muscles in the arteries, which helps reduce blood pressure. Although temporary, with regular use it has cumulative effects.

✔ **They support organ function.** Nourishing qi supports the function of all organs, and in this case, the heart and kidneys. Qi provides vitality, and blockages in qi flow decrease the heart's and kidney's abilities to function.

✔ **They improve circulation.** In Chapter 3, we tell you that where qi goes, blood follows. In addition, the nervous system controls constriction of arteries; acupressure and reflexology stimulate the regulatory function of the nervous system, causing improved blow flow and heart function.

✔ **They decrease inflammation.** Inflammation attracts cells and cholesterol that form plaque on the artery walls, decreasing blood flow. Acupressure and reflexology can't directly reduce atherosclerosis, but they can help reduce inflammation.

When air won't flow free

A variety of factors can negatively affect your breathing. Check out the following list for details:

✔ **Smoking:** Perhaps the most obvious cause of breathing problems is smoking. In addition to causing lung cancer, smoking also damages your lungs and makes it tougher to breathe deeply and effectively. When you quit smoking, the benefits to your lungs begin almost immediately. You actually begin to breathe better (and experience reduced blood pressure) within minutes after puffing that last cigarette.

✔ **Pollution:** Pollutants other than cigarette smoke also affect your lungs and make breathing more difficult. These pollutants can be found in smog, exhaust fumes from large trucks, the materials emitted from smokestacks, and numerous other sources.

✔ **Asthma and allergies:** Quite a few medical conditions can affect your breathing. Asthma is one of the biggest culprits. Asthma is a chronic inflammatory condition affecting the lungs — and it can be life-threatening in some cases. There are also great herbal remedies for treating the symptoms of allergies, and acupuncture is helpful to many people.

✔ **Serious medical conditions:** On the serious end of the spectrum, heavy-duty health problems like lung cancer, emphysema, and tuberculosis can inflict serious damage on the lungs, in some cases, making breathing virtually impossible without the help of a respiratory or oxygen tube.

✔ **Temporary conditions:** Temporary conditions like the flu, bronchitis, and common colds can also compromise your lungs' ability to perform at peak capacity. In addition, allergies can often have a negative impact on your breathing.

By using acupressure and reflexology techniques that encourage better breathing, you help your lungs perform to the best of their ability, and you allow your entire body to enjoy the benefits of an ample supply of vital oxygen. These techniques help in the following ways:

✔ They open airway passages.

✔ They relieve constrictive tension in the chest.

✔ They deepen breathing patterns.

✔ They improve cell function — qi flow nourishes every cell in the body.

✔ They improve immune function by balancing qi throughout the body.

A Healing Session to Keep Your Ticker Tockin'

The heart routine in this chapter uses the points in Figures 15-1 and 15-2, which are described in Table 15-1, to help you keep your heart healthy and beating strong. Learning and finding these points before you do the routine will help you be confident and correct in your session.

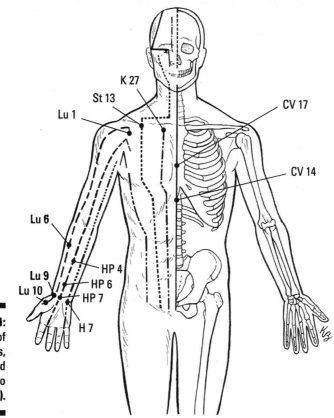

Figure 15-1:
Acupoints of
the arms,
hands, and
upper torso
(front).

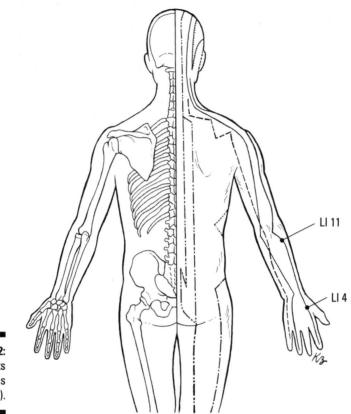

Figure 15-2:
Acupoints
of the arms
(back).

Table 15-1		Acupoints to Benefit the Heart	
Point Abbreviation	**Name of Point**	**How You Find It**	**Benefits**
H 7	Spirit Gate	On the palm side of the wrist, in the crease of the wrist, directly under the little finger.	Nourishes all aspects of the heart: It's used for all heart syndromes and diseases, arrhythmias, palpitations, and angina pectoris as well as hypertension.

Point Abbreviation	Name of Point	How You Find It	Benefits
HP 4	Crevice Gate	On the palm side of the arm, halfway between the wrist and the elbow, and then one chon toward the wrist. This point is in line with the middle finger.	Used for rheumatic heart disease, angina pectoris, chest and heart pain, palpitations, and fast heartbeat.
HP 6	Inner Gate	On the palm side of the hand, in the middle of the arm, three finger-widths above the wrist crease.	Regulates, strengthens, and protects the heart. Used for cardiac and chest pain, rheumatic heart disease, palpitations, and anxiety.
HP 7	Great Mound	Go to the palm side of the wrist crease and find the point halfway between the inside and outside of the wrist.	Regulates and clears fire in the heart; used for palpitations, chest pain, and anxiety.
LI 11	Crooked Pond	At the top of the elbow crease, on the edge of the joint.	Facilitates qi and blood flow; used for hypertension.
K 27	Shu Mansion	Under the collarbone in the depression next to the breastbone.	Tonifies the kidneys, maintaining fluid balance. Opens the chest, and is used for chest pain, chest tightness, palpitations, and anxiety.
CV 14	Great Palace Gate	Two chon below the bottom of your breastbone in the midline of the body; hold gently.	Good for chest pain, palpitations, and anxiety.
CV 17	Upper Sea of Qi	In the center of the breastbone, halfway between the top and bottom, and then down one chon.	Used to reduce palpitations and cardiac pain.

Using this routine helps your heart maintain strong function, supplying life-giving blood to all organs and tissues in the body. If you have a specific concern, you can shorten the routine and use only the points that address that concern. H 7 and HP 6 are key points that can be used for all conditions. Remember that heart health is often a lifestyle issue and can't be corrected without lifestyle changes. (Heart concerns are serious; don't neglect medical care!)

1. **Belly breathe while centering and grounding.**

2. **Stretch the meridians in the arms and chest by following these steps:**

   - Stand with your feet shoulder-width — or farther — apart.

   - Bend your knees slightly.

   - Breathe in while raising your arms, palms down, to shoulder level.

   - Continue breathing in, and spread your arms backward at shoulder level while rotating your hands palms up.

   - Reach your thumbs toward the floor behind you.

   - Exhale and relax, bringing your arms back to your side.

   - Repeat three times.

3. **Start with either arm, and use alternating pressure for full points or sustained pressure for empty points (refer to Chapter 4 for a refresher). Work each of the following points for 1 to 3 minutes:**

   - Using one meridian at a time, press HP 4, HP 6, HP 7, H 7, and LI 11. Repeat this entire sequence two or three times, until you establish an *even flow* (the points feel mostly equal to each other in fullness and tenderness).

   - Press K 27 bilaterally.

   - Press both CV 14 and CV 17 together and hold for 3 minutes.

4. **Relax by lying quietly and slowing down your breathing, which also slows the mind.**

   Allow the qi to respond to your directions in the routine by giving it time to fully balance. You may notice warmth or tingling through your body, especially in your chest.

If you have time, follow this routine with the corresponding reflexology routine for the heart and lungs, which we include later in this chapter in the section "Reflexology: Massaging the Heart and Lungs Through the Feet."

A Healing Session to Open Your Airways

The points in Table 15-2 can be like a breath of fresh air for people whose respiratory system isn't running as smoothly as they'd like. If the directions are confusing, check Chapter 3 for a refresher on using chon. You can find the points for the helpful breathing routine that follows in Figures 15-1 and 15-2, earlier in the chapter, as well as Figure 15-3, in this section.

Table 15-2		Acupoints for Respiratory Health	
Point Abbreviation	*Name of Point*	*How You Find It*	*Benefits*
Lu 1	Central Treasury	This point is located on your rib cage one chon down from where your arm meets your chest wall. Use your thumbs to press this point toward the breastbone.	Good for chest fullness, pneumonia, tuberculosis, asthma, bronchitis, wheezing, and shortness of breath.
Lu 6	Collection Hole	On the palm side of the arm, halfway between the wrist and elbow, and then one chon toward the elbow. This point is in line with the thumb.	Used for asthma, coughs, and acute lung diseases.
Lu 9	Great Abyss	On the palm side of the hand, under the thumb, in the wrist crease.	Relieves cough, asthma, bronchitis, tuberculosis, and emphysema.
Lu 10	Fish Border	On the palm surface of the hand, halfway between the outside of the wrist and the first joint of the thumb in the fleshy part of the pad. It will be very tender.	Used for pneumonia, asthma, fever, chest and back pain, and shortness of breath.
K 27	Shu Mansion	Under the collarbone in the depression next to the breastbone.	Alleviates asthma, bronchitis, chest pain and congestion, cough, shortness of breath, allergies of the chest, and difficulties breathing.

(continued)

Table 15-2 *(continued)*

Point Abbreviation	Name of Point	How You Find It	Benefits
St 13	Qi Door	Just underneath the collarbone, halfway between the breast-bone and the point of the shoulder.	Good for chest heaviness, short-ness of breath, bronchitis, cough-ing, and diaphragm spasms.
LI 4*	Union Valley	In the webbing where the index finger and the thumb meet. If you close your finger and thumb, you find it at the bottom of the crease. You can pinch this point between your index finger and thumb.	Relieves allergic asthma, bronchitis, and allergies asso-ciated with hay fever, sneezing, and itchy eyes.
LI 11	Crooked Pond	At the top of the elbow crease, on the edge of the joint.	Use for bronchitis, chest pain, allergies, hives, and itching.
LI 20	Welcome Fragrance	Just outside the nostril, pressing up into the cheekbone.	Good for stuffy nose and sinusitis.
St 3	Great Bone Hole	Slide your finger from the outside of the nostril along the cheek-bone to the lowest point of the bone, directly in line with the pupil of the eye. Press up into the bone from underneath.	Good for sinusitis, stuffy nose, allergy-related burning eyes, and sneezing.
B 2	Bright Light	At the inner corner of your eyebrow, press-ing into the orbit bone.	Use for allergy headaches, sinus pain, and hay fever.
CV 17	Upper Sea of Qi	Exact center of the breastbone, halfway between the top and bottom.	Relieves asthma, cough, bronchitis, chest pain and dis-tention, and short-ness of breath. Helps heal tuberculosis.

Never use this point during pregnancy.

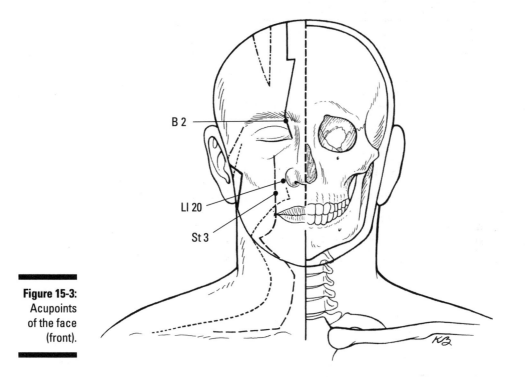

Figure 15-3:
Acupoints
of the face
(front).

Although balancing the qi in the chest and lungs benefits all breathing conditions, you may want to focus on something specific. This routine helps you with both the general and the specific:

1. **Belly breathe while centering and grounding.**

2. **Stretch the meridians in the arms and chest by following the process described in Step 2 of the preceding section.**

3. **Start with either arm, and use alternating pressure for full points or sustained pressure for empty points. (See Chapter 4 for explanations on techniques.) Work each point for 1 to 3 minutes.**

   • Use one meridian at a time and press Lu 1, Lu 6, Lu 9, and Lu 10.

   • Repeat with the other arm.

   • Use a bilateral approach and press K 27 and St 13.

- Use one meridian at a time to press LI 4 and LI 11.

- Repeat on the other arm.

- If you're having trouble breathing due to a clogged nose or sinus problems, use a bilateral approach and press LI 20, St 3, and B 2. Otherwise, you can skip these points.

4. **If you want to specifically focus on one type of chest problem, you can hold any combination of the following points:**

   - **Asthma:** Lu 1, Lu 6, Lu 9, Lu 10, K 27

   - **Allergy:** K 27, LI 4, St 3, B 2

   - **Bronchitis:** Lu 1, Lu 9, K 27, St 13

   - **Emphysema:** Lu 1, Lu 6, Lu 9, K 27, St 13

   - **Sinusitis:** St 3, LI 20

5. **End by pressing CV 17 for 3 minutes with sustained pressure.**

6. **Relax, by lying or sitting quietly, and let the qi flow rebalance as it responds to your session.**

   You may want to spend this time meditating or breathing deeply and evenly, calming your body and mind.

If you want, you can follow this routine with the chest-relieving reflexology routine for the heart and lungs (see the next section).

Reflexology: Massaging the Heart and Lungs Through the Feet

Reflexology is thought to work by stimulating the nervous system, which ultimately controls body functions. As we discuss earlier in this chapter, the nervous system is the master controller of heart and lung function. Stimulating the corresponding reflex areas on the foot or hands helps balance the nervous system's control, thereby calming and strengthening the heart and opening airways into the lungs.

Use the following routine to address heart and lung problems with reflexology — refer to Chapter 4 for information on how to perform the techniques:

1. **Wash and dry your feet.**

2. **If you haven't already stretched and performed deep breathing exercises, do some deep belly breathing now.**

3. **Sit in a chair or on a bed and cross your leg so that you can hold your foot in your lap.**

4. **Roll your foot back and forth in your hand, loosening up any restrictions.**

5. **Use horizontal stripping to further open the zones of your foot.**

6. **Find the reflex zones for the heart, lungs, and chest on your reflexology map in Figure 15-4.**

   These areas are in the ball of the foot. The lungs are found on both feet, but the heart has a reflex point only on the left foot, off the outside of the lung reflex area.

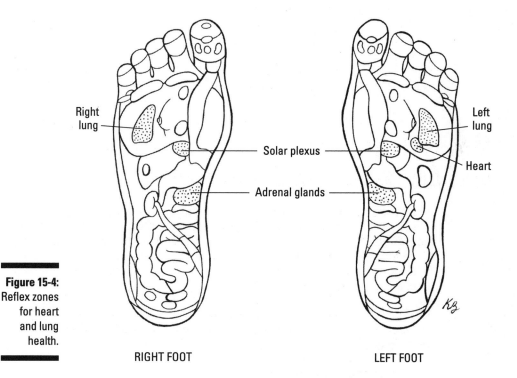

Figure 15-4:
Reflex zones
for heart
and lung
health.

RIGHT FOOT   LEFT FOOT

7. **Thumb-walk, looking for any nodules, soreness, or crackling sounds.**

   Use circular motions to work out the tension.

8. **End with thumb-walking and circular motions to the solar plexus and the adrenals to stimulate smooth qi flow.**

9. **Repeat with the other foot.**

10. **Relax while lying quietly and let the nervous system fully integrate the stimulation you have provided.**

    You may notice that you're breathing more deeply and/or your heart is beating more slowly.

Part IV

Addressing Specific Needs and Concerns

The 5th Wave · By Rich Tennant

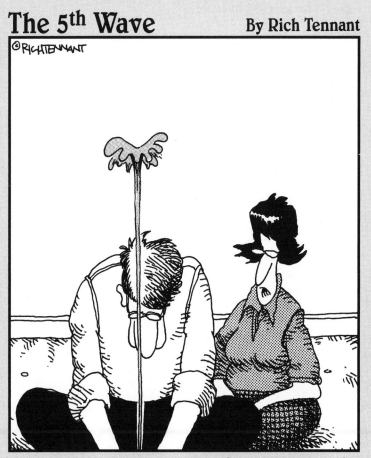

"I would use less pressure when massaging the baby's abdomen."

In this part . . .

Depending upon your specific situation, you probably have specific concerns or problems that are a high priority. In this part, we address the problems faced by particular groups of people.

Perhaps you're facing an age-related condition: a problem plaguing your baby or child, or something that you're dealing with because of the stage of life you're in. No matter what your age, we've got you covered.

If you're a female reader, you face your own specific group of problems and challenges, ranging from monthly pain to the discomfort associated with pregnancy and labor. You'll be relieved to know that we include several helpful treatments and tips in this part especially for you.

Do you dread cold and flu season? Are you constantly battling chronic conditions? Then you won't want to miss the helpful treatments in this part that target those problems.

No matter who you are or what problems you have, we think you'll find something just for you in this part.

Chapter 16

Age-Related Treatments

As most people are painfully aware, everyone's body changes (and not always in ways you like) as you age. Your physical challenges and health concerns as youngsters are totally different from those you face as seniors. Specific pains and problems tend to plague those in the midlife years, for example, whereas these conditions may not be a concern for younger people.

Bodywork isn't necessarily a one-size-fits-all type of thing. Sure, everyone is likely to get benefits of some sort from just about any of the techniques practiced in acupressure and reflexology. Bodywork is a fantastic remedy because, unlike medications or more stressful treatment approaches, its techniques are gentle enough for almost everyone. (In the case of someone who's extremely delicate or frail, obviously you proceed with caution.) To reap the maximum rewards, however, make an effort to spend some time on the techniques geared specifically to the concerns that are common among people in your age group (or that of the loved one you want to help).

In this chapter, we touch on some techniques geared to people of specific age groups, from infants to seniors and everyone in between.

Just for Kids

True, babies and kids aren't yet old enough to face the litany of aches and pains that adults must deal with (often resulting from years of hard work, overexertion, and bad habits). But as any parent knows, babies and children tend to have a laundry list of aches and pains all their own: teething, digestive discomfort, earaches, and so on.

Also, despite the fact that they often seem to have endless supplies of it, their energy isn't always flowing as well as it should. Kids need all that energy because their bodies have lots of hard work to do. We're not talking just about all that running, jumping, and playing. On a daily basis, their bodies are continuously changing, maturing, and getting stronger. Handling these growing pains isn't easy, and kids need all the help they can get.

Infants and toddlers

Nothing is worse for a parent than feeling helpless while your child struggles with physical discomfort. Acupressure can be an effective way for you to help with some of the simple aches and pains of growing, but it has its own challenges. For one thing, babies are small, and finding points can be hard. Don't worry; finding the general area still stimulates healing qi. Your child always benefits from calming and nourishing qi, whatever the situation is.

You can massage the acupoints that we introduce throughout this section (see Figure 16-1 to locate them) any time your baby is having discomfort — in a car, at the park, or anywhere. When you want to use a full routine, the perfect time is while bathing, massaging, dressing for bed, or nursing your baby.

Infants respond quickly to acupressure, so shorter sessions of 10 or 15 minutes are all you need.

Try the following routine with the points throughout the following sections, and you're likely to see a much happier and more content baby:

1. **Gently squeeze and release your baby's arms and legs.**

   You don't need to stretch an infant; babies are pretty loose already.

2. **Find the acupoints you want to use (see Tables 16-1, 16-2, and 16-3) and massage them gently, using circular motions with very light pressure.**

   You can use the points in any order or combination, or on any part of the body. Just try to incorporate all the points for the condition you're caring for. You can also use points from different tables in this chapter as needed.

   Be careful with pressure. With infants, light soothing massage over the point is perfect. Also, don't spend too much time on any point. The most you need to spend is 30 seconds, because children respond more quickly than adults.

3. **When you finish, continue with your normal routine.**

   Your baby should be calmer and more comfortable.

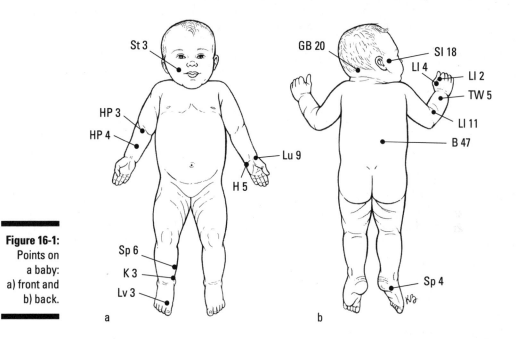

Figure 16-1:
Points on
a baby:
a) front and
b) back.

St 3

HP 3

HP 4

Lu 9

H 5

Sp 6

K 3

Lv 3

a

GB 20

SI 18

LI 4

LI 2

TW 5

LI 11

B 47

Sp 4

b

Overcoming colic

Colic is a condition that affects many babies. According to the Mayo Clinic, colic is defined as "crying for more than three hours a day, three days a week for more than three weeks in an otherwise healthy, well fed baby." The crying usually happens at the same time each day, is intense, and the baby tightens his muscles in pain. It can start within a month after birth and is usually resolved by 3 months.

No one knows the cause of colic. Food allergies or lactose intolerance were thought to be the cause, but many children with colic don't have these conditions. Other culprits are thought to be immature digestive systems, immature nervous systems, or abnormal bowel flora causing excessive gas. After extensive research, no one knows why some babies have colic and others don't. Often conditions such as gastric reflux and food allergies are misdiagnosed as colic, which is too bad because even though colic has no real treatment, you can treat these other conditions.

Colic can be an extremely stressful and exhausting experience for both baby and parent. Even though you can't treat colic, parents find little tricks to help, like bouncing the baby or swaddling the baby very tightly. Acupressure may also help, so try focusing on the points in Table 16-1 to help relieve the pain of colic.

Table 16-1	Points for Soothing Colic	
Point Abbreviation	*Name of Point*	*How You Find It*
LI 2	Second Interval	This point is on the outside of the index finger, on the metacarpal-phalanges (MCP) joint where the finger meets the hand.
B 47	Will's Chamber	This spot is on the back, halfway between the hipbone and rib cage, in the muscle just off the spine.
K 3	Great Ravine	Go to the highest point of the inner ankle-bone, and slide backward halfway to the Achilles tendon.
HP 3	Crooked Marsh	This point is in the crease of the elbow, in line with the middle finger, on the little-finger side of the biceps tendon.
Lv 3	Great Rushing	Go to the big toe, slide along the webbing between the big and second toes on the top of the foot. Press on an indent where the two metatarsal bones come closer together.

Reducing teething pain

Teething can be a painful experience for a baby, causing the child to lose sleep and become very unhappy overall. The pain of teeth breaking through flesh can be diminished in a number of ways; you can rub ice cubes, clove oil, or other pain-numbing substances on the gums, or even just apply pressure, as a child does when chewing on a teething ring. Acupressure and reflexology can also take the edge off by sedating the nervous system and by releasing pain-relieving endorphins. Table 16-2 shows points that can help alleviate some of the pain associated with teething.

Table 16-2	Points for Relieving Teething Pain	
Point Abbreviation	*Name of Point*	*How You Find It*
TW 5	Outer Gate	Three fingers above the wrist crease on the outside of the forearm.
Lu 9	Great Abyss	On the palm side of the hand, under the thumb, in the wrist crease.
LI 4	Union Valley	On the webbing where the index finger and the thumb meet. You can pinch this point between your index finger and thumb.

Point Abbreviation	Name of Point	How You Find It
LI 11	Crooked Pond	In the top of the elbow crease, on the edge of the joint.
St 3	Great Bone Hole	Slide your finger from the outside of the nostril along the cheekbone to the lowest point of the bone, and press up into the bone from underneath.
SI 18	Cheekbone Hole	Continue to slide up the cheekbone from St 3 to the depression before the ear.

Soothing the way to sleep

For small babies (and their parents), sleep can seem like an elusive luxury. Babies lose sleep for a number of reasons, such as overstimulation or even tummy aches and pains. Reflexology and acupressure calm and sedate fussy babies by smoothing turbulent qi flow. They can help reduce pain by increasing levels of endorphins — and these pain-reducing neurotransmitters are also effective sleep aids. Because lullabies and teddy bears can work only a limited number of miracles, Table 16-3 shows some points you may want to try to help your baby (and you) get a good night's sleep. (If you're not sure what a chon is, check out Chapter 3.)

Table 16-3	Points for Inducing Sleep	
Point Abbreviation	Name of Point	How You Find It
GB 20	Wind Pool	This point is along the ridge of the occipital bone, halfway between the ear and spine, and between the two muscles that come together.
Sp 4	Grandfather-Grandson	This point is on the side of the inside of the foot, one chon behind the base of the big toe. Find the bone in the arch of the foot, hook your finger into the arch from underneath, and press upward.
Sp 6	Three Yin Crossing	This point is two chon (three finger-widths) above the inner anklebone along the back of the tibia.

(continued)

Table 16-3 *(continued)*		
Point Abbreviation	*Name of Point*	*How You Find It*
H 5	Connecting Palace	This point is on the palm side of the hand, under the little finger, one chon above the crease of the wrist.
HP 4	Crevice Gate	On the palm side of the arm, go halfway between the wrist and the elbow, and then one chon toward the wrist, in line with the middle finger.

Older kids

Imagine that your child is (fortunately) past the colicky stage and firmly entrenched in early childhood. Although teething and other infant concerns are no longer issues, kids of this age have their own problems to deal with, primarily in the form of boo-boos. One advantage: Older children have the verbal skills to express their pain, discomfort, and unhappiness (and trust us, they will!), so employing bodywork techniques to ease the pain can be a lifesaver. Figure 16-2 shows some helpful points to use on children, and Table 16-4 describes each point individually. (If you're not sure what a chon is, refer to Chapter 3.)

Although bodywork can be effective for handling minor, routine aches and pains, any serious/sudden pain or severe injuries should be treated by a medical professional.

Table 16-4	**Points for Easing Minor Childhood Ailments**		
Point Abbreviation	*Name of Point*	*How You Find It*	*Benefits*
Lu 1	Central Treasury	On the rib cage, one chon down from where the arm meets the chest wall. Use your thumbs to press this point toward the breastbone.	Reduces hiccups and relieves congestion from colds.
LI 4	Union Valley	On the webbing where the index finger and the thumb meet. If you close your finger and thumb, you'll find the point at the bottom of the crease. You can pinch the point between your index finger and thumb.	Relieves earaches, colds, and congestion.

Point Abbre-viation	Name of Point	How You Find It	Benefits
LI 11	Crooked Pond	On the muscle under and slightly behind the earlobe.	Reduces fevers, relieves colds, and helps immune-system function.
H 7	Spirit Gate	On the palm side of the wrist, in the crease of the wrist, directly under the little finger.	Soothes bad dreams, calms the system, and helps with insomnia.
HP 6	Inner Gate	On the palm side of the hand, in the middle of the arm, three finger-widths above the wrist crease.	Soothes bad dreams, relieves hiccups, and calms nervous anxiety. This point also relieves nausea and vomiting.
K 27	Shu Mansion	Under the collarbone in the depression next to the breastbone.	Relieves hiccups, and alleviates colds, congestion, and asthma.
CV 17	Upper Sea of Qi	This point is in the exact center of the breastbone, halfway between top and bottom, and then slightly lower.	Calms the system, reduces conges tion, and relieves hiccups.
TW 21	Ear Gate	In front and at the top of the tragus (the little cartilage flap that covers the opening to the ear canal).	Relieves earaches.
SI 19	Hearing Palace	Directly in front of the tragus.	Relieves earaches.
GB 2	Hearing Meeting	This point is in front of the ear, directly below SI 19.	Relieves earaches.
TW 5	Outer Gate	Two chon above the wrist crease on the outside of the hand.	Relieves earaches, reduces fevers andchills, and helps overcome all illnesses.

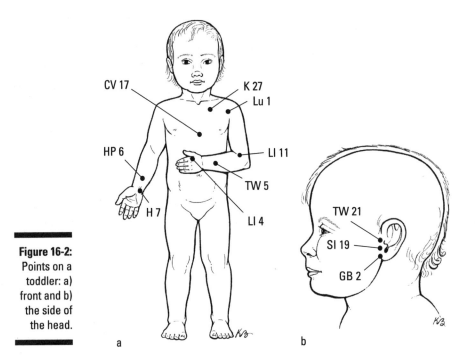

Figure 16-2:
Points on a
toddler: a)
front and b)
the side of
the head.

Older kids are easier to work with than infants in some ways and more difficult in other ways. They're a little larger and closer to adult proportions, so
finding the points is a bit easier. On the other hand, they move around a lot
and don't have a long attention span for receiving acupressure.

When you work with toddlers, keep the pressure light, and incorporate circular massage on the points for added relaxation. Don't worry too much about
finding the exact spot; you're still stimulating healing qi.

Keep the sessions short. Fewer than 20 minutes is best for your child's attention span and keeps him from overstimulating his qi.

As with babies, bedtime is an ideal time to use acupressure. If your child is
too sick or grouchy to play games, skip Steps 1 and 2. Otherwise, follow this
routine:

1. **Play a deep-breathing game with your child (refer to Chapter 2 for
   more on this warm-up exercise).**

   Kids are pretty good at belly breathing, because they do it all the time.
   But encourage your child with a "Simon Says" or "Follow the Leader"
   type of game.

2. **Play a stretching game with your child.**

   Kids are pretty loose, too, but it never hurts them to do a good stretch. Again, make stretching a game, and encourage your child to stretch her whole body. (*Stretching For Dummies,* by LaReine Chabut and published by Wiley, has some great stretches that most kids love doing.)

3. **Because all the points you use in this routine are on the front and side of the body, have your child lie on her back (face up).**

4. **Pick your points from Table 16-4, according to what your child needs.**

   If your child needs some of the points from the infant routines (refer to Tables 16-1, 16-2, and 16-3, as well as Figure 16-1), don't hesitate to use them; they work for all ages.

   Using the bilateral method or working one meridian at a time, and applying sustained pressure to tonify empty points and pulsating pressure to disperse full points, press the points that are closest to the head or chest first, ending with the points on the arms.

5. **Read your child a story or give her a bedtime cuddle as she integrates the energy from the session.**

Reflexology for youngsters of all ages

Foot reflexology works great for kids as long as they aren't too ticklish. If they are, you may have to skip the healthy benefits of reflex stimulation until they outgrow the tickles.

In general, light, narrow (finger-width) touch is more ticklish than steady, broad (whole-hand) touch, so opt for the latter. Using the pad at the base of your thumb to rub the entire foot is an overall tonic.

This routine works well for infants, toddlers, and older kids, and you can do it while washing them in a bath:

1. **Warm up by using the pads of your thumbs or the pads at the base of your thumbs to massage the entire foot gently and thoroughly.**

2. **Start by thumb-walking the chest and lung points in the ball of the foot (see Figure 16-3) to help clear congestion.**

   Feel for nodules, crystals, and sore spots to use circular motions on.

3. **Thumb-walk the areas for the ears and sinuses.**

   Ear points are located at the base of the second and third toes, and the sinus points are located on the toe pad. Pull, squeeze, and roll the toes from the base to the point, using circular motions on any nodules or sore spots. Work in as many directions as you can.

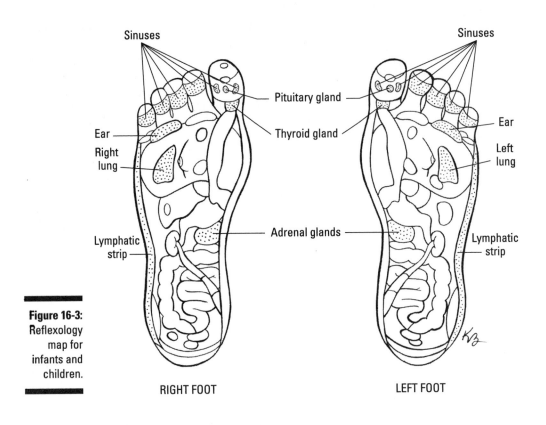

Sinuses

Sinuses

Pituitary gland

Thyroid gland

Ear

Ear

Right lung

Left lung

Lymphatic strip

Adrenal glands

Lymphatic strip

Figure 16-3:
Reflexology map for infants and children.

RIGHT FOOT

LEFT FOOT

4. **Thumb-walk the lymphatic strip along the outside edge of the foot to help clear infection and stimulate the immune system.**

   As always, use circular motions to dispel any soreness or nodules.

5. **Use circular motion on the pituitary, thyroid, and adrenal glands.**

   You can promote sleep by helping balance the endocrine glands, especially the pituitary, thyroid, and adrenal glands. You can find the pituitary point on the big toe and the thyroid point at the base of the big toe. The points for the adrenal glands, which regulate the stress response, are just below the ball of the foot on the inside of the arch. Spending extra time on both these places can help promote a good night's sleep.

6. **If you want to address any other problem areas, use circular motion or thumb-walk those reflex areas.**

7. **End by holding the feet with your whole hands, transmitting good thoughts for good dreams.**

Midlife Issues

If you ask us, midlife gets a bad rap. The pessimistic types tend to act as though their life (at least, the fun part) is pretty much history when they reach this point. Nothing could be further from the truth. As the word *midlife* implies, half your life is still ahead of you, filled with all sorts of exciting possibilities. Sure, some parts of your body may look and feel different from the way they did when you were a teenager, but that's not always a bad thing. Remember acne and that awkward growth spurt that plagued your junior-high days?

For all its good points, the midlife period admittedly can come with its share of stress, exhaustion, and emotional highs and lows. The typical midlife crisis is a roller coaster of hormonal changes and shifting life issues. Transitions are never easy; focusing on the points that we use in this section (illustrated in Figures 16-4, 16-5, and 16-6, and explained in Table 16-5) can help you deal with these challenges.

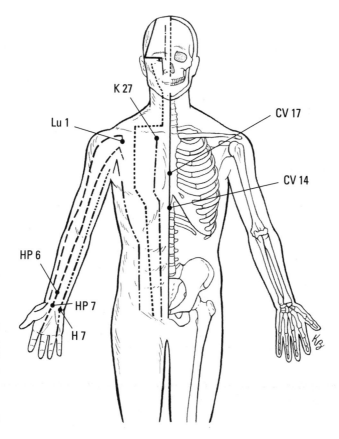

Figure 16-4:
Acupoints of the upper torso and arms (front).

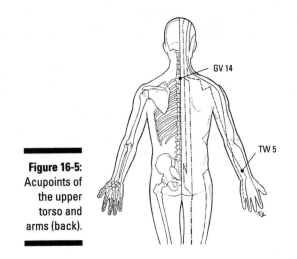

Figure 16-5:
Acupoints of
the upper
torso and
arms (back).

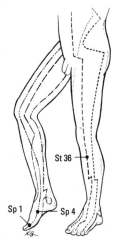

Figure 16-6:
Acupoints
of the legs
and feet
(front/side).

Table 16-5		Points for Easing Emotions of Mid-Lifers	
Point Abbreviation	**Name of Point**	**How You Find It**	**Benefits**
K 27	Shu Mansion	Under the collarbone in the depression next to the breastbone.	Relieves disorientation, anxiety, and irritability.
H 7	Spirit Gate	On the palm side of the wrist, in the crease of the wrist directly under the little finger.	Eases irritability, anxiety, fear, mood swings, and depression.
HP 7	Great Mound	On the palm side of the wrist, in the middle of the wrist crease.	Protects against excess stress; calms and sedates body and mind.
TW 5	Outer Gate	Two chon (three finger-widths) above the wrist crease on the outside of the hand.	Regulates excess emotions.
Sp 4	Grandfather-Grandson	On the side of the inside of the foot, one chon behind the base of the big toe. Find the bone in the arch of the foot, hook your finger into the arch from underneath, and press upward.	Relieves insomnia, depression, and restlessness.

You may also be experiencing the aches and pains of old injuries, arthritis, or chronic muscle tension from all that desk work you do. Maybe you're having trouble keeping your blood pressure low, or maybe you're experiencing other degenerative conditions. If so, acupressure and reflexology can help. Bodywork can balance immune function, stimulate healing and repair mechanisms, lower blood pressure, and reduce pain — all these things make acupressure and reflexology ideal for midlife concerns. If you identify with any of these physical concerns, look up the appropriate chapter in Part III of this book and find the routine you need.

If midlife problems have you tired and stressed, try this routine for some much-needed relief:

1. **Belly breathe while centering and grounding (see Chapter 2).**

2. **Stretch the meridians in the arms and chest:**

   • Stand with your feet shoulder-width apart or farther.

   • Bend your knees slightly.

   • Breathe in while raising your arms to shoulder level, palms down. Continue breathing in, and spread your arms backward at shoulder-blade level while rotating your hands palms up. Reach your thumbs toward the floor behind you.

   • Exhale and relax, bringing your arms back to your side.

   • Repeat three times.

3. **Use a bilateral hold on K 27 for 1 to 3 minutes with sustained or alternating pressure.**

4. **Starting with either arm, work H 7, HP 7, and TW 5 in any order, using alternating or sustained pressure as indicated, and working each point for 1 to 3 minutes.**

5. **Repeat Step 4 with the other arm.**

6. **Bilaterally hold Sp 4 on the inside of the foot for 1 to 3 minutes.**

   This point usually is sore, so you may want to use circular motions to ease the congested qi.

7. **Relax, or follow with the supportive reflexology routine at the end of the chapter (see "Reflexology for Teens and Adults").**

For Seniors

You've left the midlife period behind and are coming to terms with your more "mature" self. These years truly are your golden years, and you should treasure all the wonderful experiences you're having.

If you find enjoyment tough to come by because your bones are achin' or you generally just feel wiped out, try a dose of acupressure or reflexology. The free movement of qi throughout your body may deliver the pain relief or the boost of energy you need. Also, when practiced on a regular basis, acupressure and reflexology may lead to less pain and better mental and physical function in the long term.

Moving qi through your body

You're never too old to support your qi and reap the rewards of a better-balanced energy flow. You can find acupressure and reflexology routines for many of the aches and pains you may be experiencing in Part III of this book. Maybe you're having a harder time resisting illness, catching everything that comes around — if so, head to Chapter 18. Or maybe you're having trouble with arthritis in your knees or with your heart — if that's you, check out Chapters 10 and 15, respectively. However, if you need more energy to pursue the things that interest you in life, this is the chapter for you. Replenishing and stimulating qi flow helps all the systems in the body and helps you find the get-up-and-go you may be looking for.

To help support your qi in your senior years, concentrate on the points illustrated in Figures 16-4, 16-5, and 16-6, earlier in this chapter, and listed in Table 16-6.

Table 16-6	**Points to Enhance Qi Flow for Strength and Vitality**		
Point Abbre-viation	**Name of Point**	**How You Find It**	**Benefits**
St 36	Three Mile Point	One chon out from the shinbone and three chon (one palm-width) below the patella.	Provides overall general strengthening.
Sp 4	Grandfather-Grandson	On the side of the inside of the foot, one chon behind the base of the big toe. Find the bone in the arch of the foot, hook your finger into the arch from underneath, and press upward.	Stimulates leg and lower-abdominal qi.
Lu 1	Central Treasury	On the rib cage, one chon down from where the arm meets the chest wall. Using your thumbs, press this point toward the breastbone.	Opens chest and improves oxygen flow.
H 7	Spirit Gate	On the palm side of the wrist, in the crease of the wrist directly under the little finger.	Reduces fatigue due to depression or anxiety.

(continued)

Table 16-6 (continued)

Point Abbreviation	Name of Point	How You Find It	Benefits
CV 17	Upper Sea of Qi	In the center of the breastbone, halfway between top and bottom, one chon lower than center. It's the connecting point for all yin meridians.	Stimulates qi, energizes the upper body, and stimulates yin flow.
GV 14	Great Hammer	At the big vertebrae where your neck meets your back. It's the connecting point for all yang meridians.	Tonifies (strengthens) and smoothes yang energy.

Use the following routine whenever you need an energy boost:

1. **Belly breathe while centering and grounding (see Chapter 2).**

2. **Stretch the meridians in the arms and chest:**

   • Stand with your feet shoulder-width apart or farther.

   • Bend your knees slightly.

   • Breathe in while raising your arms to shoulder level, palms down. Continue breathing in, and spread your arms backward at shoulder-blade level while rotating your hands palms up. Reach your thumbs toward the floor behind you.

   • Exhale and relax, bringing your arms back to your side.

   • Repeat three times.

3. **Use a bilateral hold on St 36, Sp 4, and Lu 1.**

   Use alternating or sustained pressure, and hold each point for 1 to 3 minutes.

4. **Use the "one meridian at a time" technique from Chapter 4 for H 7 on both arms.**

5. **End by holding CV 17 and GV 14 together for 3 minutes.**

6. **Relax, or follow with reflexology (see "Reflexology for Teens and Adults," later in this chapter).**

Improving memory and mental function with acupressure

One of the biggest health-related complaints among senior citizens is the memory loss they often experience to varying degrees. Memory loss can be extremely stressful and upsetting to those who suffer from it. Like all parts of the body, the brain needs smooth qi flow to function well. Memory is only one function of the brain that suffers. Along with memory loss can come confusion, anxiety, and disorientation. Fortunately specific acupoints can recharge your memory and help alleviate these other symptoms as well.

People of all ages can experience occasional memory lapses — and some people are born with a terrible memory — so this routine can be helpful for everyone, not just seniors.

Table 16-7 lists points for improving memory and overall mental function. You can locate these points in Figures 16-4 and 16-6, earlier in this chapter.

Table 16-7	Points for Improving Memory, Alertness, and Mental Function		
Point Abbre-viation	**Name of Point**	**How You Find It**	**Benefits**
Sp 1	Hidden White	On the big toe at the outer edge of the nail.	Clears thinking and helps access intelligence.
K 27	Shu Mansion	Under the collarbone in the depression next to the breastbone.	Relieves mental strain and fatigue, and eases disorientation.
H 7	Spirit Gate	On the palm side of the wrist, in the crease of the wrist directly under the little finger.	Improves poor memory.
HP 6	Inner Gate	On the palm side of the hand, in the middle of the arm, three finger-widths above the wrist crease.	Relieves forgetfulness.

(continued)

Table 16-7 (continued)

Point Abbreviation	Name of Point	How You Find It	Benefits
CV 14	Great Palace Gate	Two chon below the bottom of the breastbone in the midline of the body. Hold this point gently.	Relieves chest pain, palpitations, and anxiety.
CV 17	Upper Sea of Qi	In the center of the breastbone, halfway between top and bottom, and then one chon lower. It's the connecting point for all yin meridians.	Stimulates qi, energizes the upper body, and stimulates yin flow.

The following routine can help boost memory and mental function. For all the points, use sustained pressure to tonify an empty point, or pulsating pressure to disperse a full point. Hold each point for 1 to 3 minutes.

1. **Belly breathe while centering and grounding.**

2. **Stretch the meridians in the arms and chest:**

   • Stand with your feet shoulder-width apart or farther.

   • Bend your knees slightly.

   • Breathe in while raising your arms to shoulder level, palms down. Continue breathing in, and spread your arms backward at shoulder-blade level while rotating your hands palms up. Reach your thumbs toward the floor behind you.

   • Exhale and relax, bringing your arms back to your side.

   • Repeat three times.

3. **Use bilateral holds on Sp 1 and K 27.**

4. **Starting with either arm, use one meridian at a time, and hold H 7 and HP 6.**

5. **Repeat Step 3 with the other arm.**

6. **End by holding CV 14 with CV 17 for 3 to 5 minutes for a calm mind and body.**

7. **Relax, or follow with reflexology (see the next section).**

Reflexology for Teens and Adults

You can use reflexology to address key organs and glands to relieve stress, worry, and overactive emotions; support qi; and improve memory and overall mental function. The organs involved are the lungs and heart. The key endocrine glands are the pituitary, pineal, thyroid, and adrenal glands.

Here's a reflexology routine designed with the needs of teens and adults in mind:

1. **Wash and dry your feet.**

2. **If you haven't already stretched and performed deep-breathing exercises, do some deep belly breathing now (refer to Chapter 3).**

3. **Sit in a chair or on a bed, and cross your leg so that you can hold one foot in your lap.**

4. **Roll your foot back and forth in your hand, loosening any restrictions.**

5. **Use horizontal stripping (refer to Chapter 4) to open the zones of your foot further.**

6. **Find the reflex zones for the heart, lungs, and chest on the reflexology map in Figure 16-7.**

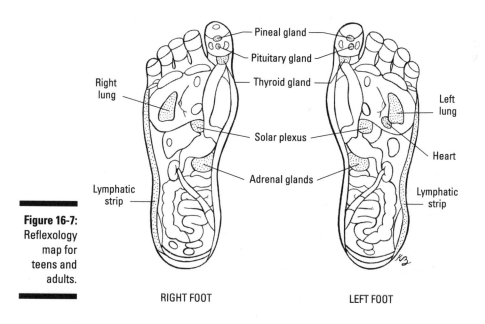

Pineal gland

Pituitary gland

Right lung

Thyroid gland

Left lung

Solar plexus

Heart

Adrenal glands

Lymphatic strip

Lymphatic strip

Figure 16-7: Reflexology map for teens and adults.

RIGHT FOOT

LEFT FOOT

These areas are in the ball of the foot. The lung zones are on both feet, but the heart has a reflex point only on the left foot, off the outside of the lung point.

7. **Thumb-walk, looking for any nodules, soreness, or crackling sounds, and use circular motions to work out tension.**

8. **Stimulate the endocrine glands by using circular motions.**

   You can find the pineal and pituitary reflex points on the big toe, and the thyroid reflex point at the base of the big toe. The reflex points for the adrenal glands, which regulate the stress response, are just below the ball of the foot on the inside of the arch.

9. **End with thumb-walking and make circular motions on the solar-plexus point in the center of the foot and on the lymphatic strip on the outside edge of the foot.**

10. **Repeat Steps 3 through 9 on the other foot.**

11. **Relax, breathe deeply, and allow qi to flow through the organs and glands you have stimulated.**

    You may feel warmth, tingling, or a sense of opening as qi moves.

Chapter 17

Especially for Women

• •

In This Chapter

▶ Recognizing the special needs of women

▶ Coping with cramps

▶ Keeping your moods in balance

▶ Easing the pain of labor

• •

*E*ven if you're for equal rights — and we certainly are — face it: physically, men and women are obviously very different. And that means that they each have their own specific needs for health and healing.

Women in particular have additional healing needs. They need something to help them cope with the physical pain and discomfort they face on a monthly basis, as well as the pain related to labor and childbirth, and menopause symptoms.

In addition, women can often experience problems as a result of the shifts in energy flow due to hormonal changes and imbalances.

By tailoring the healing plan in recognition of women's specific anatomical makeup, you can target their particular needs more efficiently.

We felt it was important to include a section specifically addressing women, because some common conditions affect a large number of women on a regular, predictable basis. (Men, on the other hand, tend to be plagued more by a variety of different conditions, such as those we discuss throughout other parts of this book.) In this chapter, we cover the major female-specific problems, including PMS and menstrual cramps, problems related to pregnancy/childbirth, and menopause symptoms.

Curtailing Menstrual Pain and PMS

One of the biggest pain-related concerns of women — and one they must deal with on a monthly basis for most of their lives — is the discomfort associated with their menstrual cycles. This discomfort includes not only menstrual cramps but also the irritation and mood swings associated with premenstrual syndrome (PMS). This discomfort is no minor inconvenience — for some women, these symptoms can last for a week or two out of every month. And women deal with more than physical discomfort: PMS can also affect a woman's sleep schedule and concentration and leave her totally exhausted.

From a Chinese medicine perspective, menstrual problems can result from a number of energetic factors, the most common being a condition of excess yin. (Refer to Chapter 1 for a discussion of yin and yang characteristics.) By balancing the yin and yang of the body, you can alleviate the symptoms of PMS. In this section, we help you do just that — see Figures 17-1, 17-2, and 17-3 to locate the points, and read about them in Table 17-1. If you're not sure how to measure chon, check out Chapter 3.

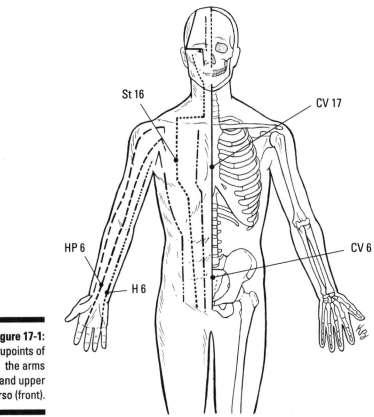

Figure 17-1:
Acupoints of the arms and upper torso (front).

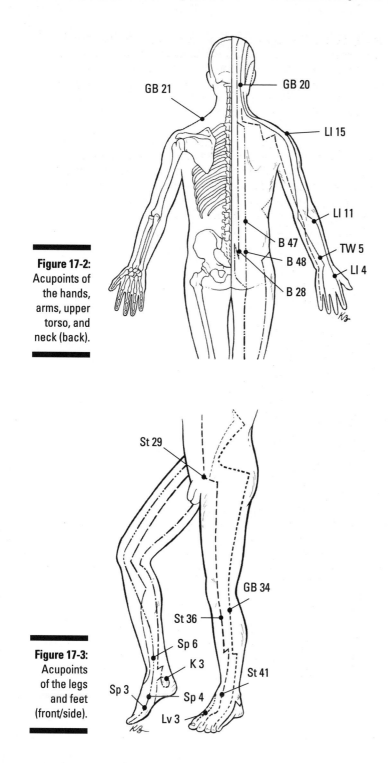

Figure 17-2:
Acupoints of the hands, arms, upper torso, and neck (back).

GB 21

GB 20

LI 15

LI 11

B 47

TW 5

B 48

LI 4

B 28

Figure 17-3:
Acupoints of the legs and feet (front/side).

St 29

GB 34

St 36

Sp 6

K 3

St 41

Sp 3

Sp 4

Lv 3

Table 17-1		Points for PMS	
Point Abbreviation	Name of Point	How You Find It	Benefits
Lv 3	Great Rushing	On the top side of the foot, go between the big and second toes; trace up the webbing between the metatarsal bones until the bones come together, forming a depression.	Use to relieve cramps of all kinds. Redirects rebellious liver qi, smoothes the flow of qi, and reduces symptoms of PMS.
Sp 4	Grandfather-Grandson	This point is on the side of the inside of the foot, one chon behind the base of the big toe. Find the bone in the arch of the foot, hook your finger into the arch from underneath, and press upward.	Good for helping with irregular menstruation.
Sp 6*	Three Yin Crossing	Three chon (four finger-widths) above the inner anklebone along the back of the tibia.	isperses stagnating Dqi, stimulates blood flow, and initiates menstruation. Can be used for irregular menstruation.
GB 34*	Yang Mound	This point is on the side of the leg, below your knee, on the head of the outer leg bone (fibula). It's slightly forward of the midline.	Reduces PMS symptoms by smoothing the flow of qi.
St 29	Return	On the outer edge of the pubic bone, two chon from the midline of the body.	Stimulates and balances the flow of qi and blood to reproductive organs, and regulates all menstrual issues.

Point Abbre-viation	Name of Point	How You Find It	Benefits
B 47	Will's Chamber	Place your hands on your waist with your fingers pointing forward and your thumbs pointing backward. Slide your thumbs toward your spine. When you hit the erector muscles, you'll find a great sore spot. It's about three chon away from the spine.	Relieves pelvic tension; reduces back pain and pelvic cramps.
CV 6	Lower Sea of Qi	Two chon below the belly button on the midline of the body.	Relieves menstrual cramps and irregular periods.
HP 6	Inner Gate	Palm side of the hand, in the middle of the arm, two chon (three finger-widths) above the wrist crease.	Calms nerves and anxiety; smoothes the flow of qi.

* Never use this point during pregnancy.

Use the following routine anytime you experience menstrual cramps:

1. **Belly breathe while centering and grounding (refer to Chapter 2).**

2. **Stretch your whole body to open the meridians involved in maintaining female health and balance (yes, that's all of them!) by following these steps:**

   • Take your arms up over your head while breathing in and stretch backward as far as you comfortably can (don't overstretch and hurt yourself!). Hold for the count of three.

   • Exhale as you bend forward, stretching your arms to the floor. Be a rag doll and hold this stretch for the count of three.

   • Inhale as you stand up; bring your arms over your head and lean to the side, exhaling while you lean. Hold.

   • Breathe in as you straighten up and repeat on the other side.

   • Repeat the whole sequence three times to fully open the meridian channels.

3. **Work the points in Table 17-1 by using sustained pressure on points that feel too empty and alternating pressure on points that feel too full.**

   Work each set of points for 1 to 3 minutes.

4. **Use bilateral holds for the following sets of points, repeating pressure on each set of points two to three times:**

   - Lv 3, Sp 4, Sp 6
   - GB 34, St 29, B 47

   Spend extra time on points that are sore or feel "needy."

5. **Hold CV 6 for 3 minutes with sustained pressure if the point is too empty or alternating pressure if the point is too full.**

   Refer to Chapter 4 for info about distinguishing between empty and full points.

6. **Alternately press HP 6 on each arm.**

7. **End with a relaxing rest, a soothing bubble bath, or some reflexology relief.**

Dulling Pregnancy and Post-Pregnancy Aches and Pains

As every woman who has ever been pregnant knows, impending motherhood is a blissful time that's often accompanied by some not-so-blissful aches and pains. In Chinese medicine, many of the minor ailments are imbalances of qi, especially in the spleen and stomach meridians where qi imbalances show up as morning sickness, food cravings, heartburn, and fatigue. On an emotional level, these meridians also demonstrate imbalance through irritability and worry. The liver, heart, and kidney meridians are also key during pregnancy, but in general, the balance of all the meridians is necessary to maintain a healthy, easy pregnancy.

Acupressure to ease pregnancy woes

Acupressure can be a great tool for assisting a happy and healthy pregnancy. It can help relieve minor aches, pains, and discomforts of carrying many extra pounds all in one place. It can help reduce excess fluid build-up in the ankles, and release nervous tension and excess excitement. It also helps balance the roller coaster of hormones and emotions and the roller coaster of your stomach during morning sickness. And don't forget the importance of smooth and adequate flow of qi to nourish all cells, including the fetus. Acupressure is great, but remember that these points powerfully affect the body and need to be used with care. Here are some tips for using acupressure during pregnancy:

- ✔ **Don't hold points for a long time — 30 seconds to 1 minute is plenty.** Holding the points for this amount of time helps avoid too many toxins being cleared from the cells at once and entering the bloodstream in one big rush. Toxins in the bloodstream can enter the baby, stressing both mommy and baby. Although removing toxins is important, slower is better in this situation.

- ✔ **Don't press the points deeply** — pregnancy is a time when everything is extra sensitive, points can be more painful as well, and the effects can be more dramatic because the body is highly tuned to react. So remember that less is more.

- ✔ **Make the sessions short — 20 minutes is plenty.** The goal is to stimulate change, but you don't want the body to do too much at one time.

- ✔ **Avoid using acupressure and reflexology when a pregnancy is fragile.** At this time a mother needs all the qi she has to sustain the pregnancy.

  Most reflexologists believe that using reflexology is safe even in fragile pregnancies because it supports the direction in which qi is needed rather than redirecting it. However, if you aren't professionally trained, avoiding both reflexology and acupressure is wise.

- ✔ **Never use the points that we list in Table 17-2 during pregnancy.** Some of these points, such as Sp 6 and LI 4, are absolutely taboo. Others are cautionary, especially during the first trimester, but should be avoided throughout just to be safe. A practiced professional will use these points as indicated, but you need more than this book to be prepared for that level of practice.

- ✔ **Do use acupressure along with reflexology (avoiding the ankles) and gentle massage to relieve the aches and pains of pregnancy.** Just make sure you follow the precautions in this list.

Table 17-2		Points to Avoid During Pregnancy	
Point Abbre-viation	**Name of Point**	**How You Find It**	**Why You Must Avoid It**
LI 4*	Union Valley	In the webbing where the index finger and the thumb meet. If you close your finger and thumb, you'll find it at the bottom of the crease. You can pinch this point between your index finger and thumb.	Activates labor and stimulates the downward flow of energy.
Sp 6*	Three Yin Crossing	Three finger-widths above the inner anklebone along the back of the tibia.	Stimulates uterine contraction, initiates downward flow of qi, and stimulates menstruation.
St 36*	Three Mile Point	One chon out from the shinbone and three chon (one palm-width) below the patella.	Stimulates energy flow to muscles and can cause uterine contractions.
GB 34*	Yang Mound	This point is on the side of the leg, below your knee, on the head of the outer leg bone (fibula).	Can cause ligament laxity and over-stretching during the first trimester of pregnancy.
CV 6*	Lower Sea of Qi	In the depression three chon below the belly button in the midline of the body.	Can send qi out of the uterus.
GB 21*	Shoulder Well	In the top of the shoulder, half-way between the point of your shoulder and the base of your neck. In the belly of the muscle.	Can increase descending qi and may cause uterine contractions.
All points on the sacrum*			Can cause uterine contractions.

* Never use any of these points during pregnancy.

Now that we've identified the points you *shouldn't* use during pregnancy, we present some that you *should* use during pregnancy. The points in Table 17-3, which you can find in Figures 17-1, 17-2, and 17-3 earlier in the chapter and in Figure 17-4 in this section, can be effective in providing some welcome relief for the mommy-to-be.

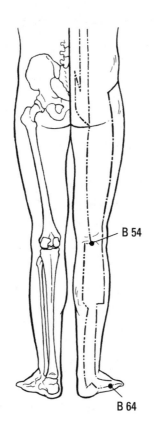

Figure 17-4:
Acupoints of
the legs and
feet (back).

B 54

B 64

Table 17-3		Points for a More Comfortable Pregnancy	
Point Abbre-viation	*Name of Point*	*How You Find It*	*Benefits*
Sp 3	Supreme Whiteness	Go to the side of the inside of the foot. Find the base of the big toe. Slide into the depression between the base of the big toe and the metatarsal bone, staying on the side of the foot.	Nourishes spleen meridian. Spleen meridian helps sustain uterus during pregnancy. Helps relieve nausea and edema.

(continued)

Table 17-3 (continued)

Point Abbreviation	Name of Point	How You Find It	Benefits
Sp 4	Grandfather-Grandson	This point is on the side of the inside of the foot, one chon behind the base of the big toe. Find the bone in the arch of the foot, hook your finger into the arch from underneath, and press upward.	Can be used for insomnia, leg pains, and constipation.
K 6	Shining Sea	On the inside of the ankle, one chon below the inside anklebone in the depression.	Relieves edema and water retention.
B 47	Will's Chamber	Place your hands on your waist with your fingers pointing forward and your thumbs pointing backward. Slide your thumbs toward your spine. When you hit the erector muscles, you'll find a great sore spot. It's about four chon away from the spine.	Relieves low backaches, sciatica, and reproductive issues.
B 54	Middle Crook	Right in the middle of the crease in the back of the knee.	Regulates and relaxes muscles. Use for low back and muscle spasms.
HP 6	Inner Gate	Palm side of the hand, in the middle of the wrist, three finger-widths above the wrist crease.	This is the point for nausea and vomiting. It's also one of the most relaxing acupuncture points and is used for both insomnia and anxiety.

Use the following routine to ease some of the aches and pains of pregnancy and prepare the woman's body for delivery. *Warning:* Be sure to follow the list of precautions when using acupressure in pregnancy and avoid all the points in Table 17-2.

1. **Start with the opening warm-up in Steps 1 and 2 of the routine for PMS relief (see the earlier section "Curtailing Menstrual Pain and PMS" for details).**

   Be sure to stretch gently and always stay within your comfort zone.

2. **To continue your warm-up, do a series of squats.**

   This stretch is one of the best you can do for pregnancy. If you can, simply spend time squatting every day. This stretch helps open your pelvis and prepare the bones, ligaments, and skin for stretching during childbirth.

3. **Use bilateral holds on the following sets of points, repeating pressure on each set of points two to three times:**

   - Sp 3, Sp 4, K 6
   - B 47, B 48, B 54

   Spend extra time on any sore points or points that feel as if they need more attention.

4. **Alternately press HP 6 on each arm.**

   You can press firmly between the two tendons that run down the arm and into the wrist. Don't worry about damaging veins or tendons; they'll move out the way of your pressure.

5. **End with a relaxing rest or some rejuvenating reflexology.**

Relief on your labor day

Although women need attention and pain relief throughout their entire pregnancy, they *really* need all the help they can get during labor. Fortunately, bodywork techniques can be effective in alleviating some of the pain associated with labor, particularly in the back. You can have your birthing partner use the points in Table 17-4, which you can locate in Figures 17-1, 17-2, and 17-3, earlier in this chapter, to ease your back pain and to support and assist your body in the delivery processes. You may notice that points that were taboo during pregnancy are great for labor to help push the baby out.

It's a good idea to have your birthing partner memorize these points. If you're supporting someone else through a birth, memorize these points in plenty of time before the event. Things start to move pretty fast, and finding maps can be impossible.

Table 17-4		Easing Labor Pains	
Point Abbreviation	**Name of Point**	**How You Find It**	**Benefits**
B 48	Bladder Vitals	Three chon to the side of the sacrum in the middle of the gluteal muscle of the buttocks. Very tender point.	Relieves back pain, and stimulates qi flow through the pelvis.
B 28	Bladder Shu	Halfway between the top and bottom of the sacrum, and halfway between the middle and outer edge.	Relieves lower and sacral back pain.
St 29	Return	On the outer edge of the pubic bone, two chon from the midline.	Stimulates and balances flow of qi to reproductive organs.
Sp 6*	Three Yin Crossing	Three finger-widths above the inner anklebone along the back of the tibia.	Regulates menstruation and labor, and stimulates uterine contractions.
LI 4*	Union Valley	In the webbing where the index finger and the thumb meet. If you close your finger and thumb, you'll find it at the bottom of the crease. You can pinch this point between your index finger and thumb.	Activates labor and stimulates a downward flow of energy.
GB 21	Shoulder Well	In the top of the shoulder, halfway between the point of your shoulder and the base of your neck. In the belly of the muscle.	Influences and stimulates the downward flow of energy.
K 3	Great Ravine	Go the highest point of the inner anklebone and slide backward, halfway to the Achilles tendon.	Relieves labor pain.

* Never use these points during pregnancy, but they're fine to use during labor!

Most acupressure routines begin with breathing and stretching exercises, but you're already using the breathing exercises you learned in your birthing classes. And forget the stretching! Your body will be stretching enough all on its own!

1. **Your partner can use the points in Table 17-4 in any order and at any time during the delivery.**

2. **Some specific points that may give you relief include the following:**

   - B 28, B 48, St 29, and K 3 are great for easing the discomfort of early labor and preparing for delivery.

   - To assist delivery, use Sp 6, LI 4, and GB 21.

3. **Rub the feet — especially after the birth.**

   Restorative reflexology works well (see the routine in Chapter 6 for optimal wellness, or use the one at the end of this chapter).

Just for new moms

Giving birth is probably the hardest thing a woman's body will ever do. Give yourself every support possible in recovering your qi; you need the energy to breastfeed and care for your baby. Breastfeeding is taxing and you may have trouble with pain or insufficient milk flow. And although labor can involve considerable pain, the discomfort doesn't end instantly after the baby is born. New moms must cope with pain, as well, which often isn't easy considering the exhausting toll of the recovery process (and, face it, babies can make it tough to get a good night's sleep).

But a mom who's tired, weak, and in pain can't fully enjoy crucial bonding moments with her new bundle of joy. So using bodywork techniques to make a new mom more comfortable can benefit both mom and baby.

Bringing qi to traumatized tissue post-delivery

For new moms, the recovery phase immediately following labor can involve considerable pain, cramping, and other discomfort. The body has to adjust to changes in hormones, restrengthen overstretched tissue, repair tears or cuts to the perineum, and recover qi. If the new mom had a C-section, she has additional challenges of repairing the surgical cuts and muscles of the abdomen and pelvic floor. For these women, the relief that bodywork provides can be a lifesaver. For the routine in this section, you can find the points in Table 17-5 and locate them in Figures 17-1, 17-2, and 17-3, earlier in this chapter.

Table 17-5		Post-Delivery Recovery Points	
Point Abbreviation	*Name of Point*	*How You Find It*	*Benefits*
CV 6	Lower Sea of Qi	In the depression three chon below the belly button in the midline of the body.	Generally uplifting, rejuvenates qi flow, and relieves general weakness. Use with care if you have had a C-section, using only finger contact with no pressure.
HP 6	Inner Gate	Palm side of the hand, in the middle of the arm, three finger-widths above the wrist crease.	Relieves postpartum depression and insomnia.
B 47	Will's Chamber	Place your hands on your waist with your fingers pointing forward and your thumbs pointing backward. Slide your thumbs toward your spine. When you hit the erector muscles, you'll find a great sore spot, about three chon away from the spine.	Relieves pelvic tension, low back pain, and genital swelling. Reduces postpartum distress.
St 36	Three Mile Point	One chon out from the shinbone and three chon (one palm-width) below the patella.	Strengthens and tones muscles, rejuvenates tissue, and helps return ligaments to normal tension.
Lv 3	Great Rushing	On the top side of the foot, go between the big and second toes; trace up the webbing between the metatarsal bones until the bones come together, forming a depression.	Relieves cramps.

To garner relief post-delivery, try the following healing routine:

1. **Belly breathe while centering and grounding.**

2. **Use the whole-body stretches from Step 2 of the routine to relieve PMS (see the earlier section "Curtailing Menstrual Pain and PMS" for details).**

3. **Stretch your chest and arm meridians by opening your arms wide and stretching them behind you as you arch your back and breathe in deeply.**

   Do these stretches two or three times.

4. **Use the following points in the following patterns, using sustained pressure on points that feel too empty and alternating pressure on points that feel too full.**

   Work each set of points for 1 to 3 minutes.

   - Hold CV 6 for 3 to 5 minutes to open the flow of energy into the Lower Sea of Qi.

   - Hold HP 6 on each arm, one meridian at a time.

   - Use bilateral holds for B 47, St 36, and Lv 3.

   - Repeat the previous two steps until the points are no longer sore or the flow feels even and smooth.

   - Finish by holding CV 6 again for 3 to 5 minutes to harmonize qi flow.

Soothing sore breasts and encouraging milk flow

Recovering from delivery can be tough enough, but the physical demands of breastfeeding can add an extra challenge for new moms. Many women have trouble starting the breastfeeding process due to congestion of chest qi or qi deficiency. Using St 13 and CV 17 can really help. And if you have trouble producing as much milk as your baby needs, St 36 and Lv 3 can stimulate qi sufficiency.

Breastfeeding may be exhausting, but it's a great way to bond with your baby. Bonus: It also helps you shed pregnancy weight fast — on average, breastfeeding burns up an extra 500 calories a day!

The specific points in Table 17-6 can help breastfeeding moms feel better. You can find the points in Figures 17-1, 17-2, and 17-3, earlier in this chapter.

Table 17-6		Points that Support Breastfeeding	
Point Abbre-viation	**Name of Point**	**How You Find It**	**Benefits**
CV 17	Upper Sea of Qi	Exact center of the breast-bone, halfway between the top and bottom, and then slightly lower.	Energizes the chest segment and opens channels of qi running through the chest.
St 16	Breast Window	On the chest, go to the middle of the collarbone and then drop one hand-width. The point is between the third and fourth rib.	Relieves breast pain, stimulates the flow of breast milk, and relieves insomnia.
St 36	Three Mile Point	One chon out from the shinbone and three chon (one palm-width) below the patella.	Use for insufficient lactation.
Lv 3	Great Rushing	On the top side of the foot, go between the big and second toes; trace up the webbing between the metatarsal bones until the bones come together, form-ing a depression.	Nourishes fluids and impacts energy flow through the breasts.
HP 6	Inner Gate	alm side of the hand, in the middle of the arm, three finger-widths above the wrist crease.	Disperses stagnant qi in the chest, and reduces anxiety and nervousness.

You can use the following routine with the points in Table 17-5 and/or Table 17-6:

1. **Belly breathe while centering and grounding.**

2. **Use the whole-body stretches from Step 2 of the routine for PMS relief (see the earlier section, "Curtailing Menstrual Pain and PMS" for details).**

3. **Stretch your chest and arm meridians by opening your arms wide and stretching them behind you as you arch your back and breathe in deeply.**

Do these stretches two or three times.

4. **Use the following points in the following patterns, using sustained pressure on points that feel too empty and alternating pressure on points that feel too full.**

   Work each set of points for 1 to 3 minutes.

   - Hold CV 17 to open energy flow into the Upper Sea of Qi.

   - Use bilateral holds for St 16, St 36, and Lv 3.

   - Hold HP 6 on each arm using one meridian at a time.

   - Repeat the previous two steps until the points are no longer sore or the flow feels even and smooth.

   - Hold CV 17 for 3 to 5 minutes to harmonize the qi flow.

     Note: If you hold points for both labor relief and breastfeeding support, drop this last step from both routines. Instead, when you're finished with both routines, hold CV 6 and CV 17 together for 3 to 5 minutes. This is a great way to end, and you can use this alternative in either routine.

5. **End with a relaxing ritual of your choice or move on to the foot reflexology routine at the end of this chapter, "Reflexology for Overall Women's Health."**

Squelching the Fires of Menopause

Menopause (and pre-menopause) can cause all sorts of uncomfortable and painful symptoms thanks to changing hormones, ranging from night sweats and hot flashes to mood swings and insomnia. Perhaps one of the most annoying symptoms of menopause, though, is the emotional roller coaster caused by fluctuating hormone levels. These up-and-down fluctuations can make life miserable for the menopausal woman (and everyone around her). Relief is here. Because qi impacts the endocrine system, acupressure can be helpful in easing the passage of menopause. We cover all those aggravating symptoms and more in this section. In the routine that follows, you use the points found in Table 17-7 and located in Figures 17-1, 17-2, and 17-3, earlier in this chapter.

Table 17-7		Acupoints for the Roller Coaster of Menopause	
Point Abbreviation	**Name of Point**	**How You Find It**	**Benefits**
GB 20	Wind Pool	Along the ridge of your occipital bone, halfway between your ear and spine; between the two muscles that come together.	Relieves hot flashes, and reduces stress and irritability.
LI 11	Crooked Pond	At the top of the elbow crease, on the edge of the joint.	Relieves hot flashes.
H 6	Yin Cleft	On the palm side of the arm, one palm-width (four chon) above the wrist crease in line with the baby finger.	Relieves night sweats, reduces anxiety, and relieves irritability.
Lv 3	Great Rushing	Go to the top of the foot to the big toe and the second toe; trace up between the bones until the bones meet.	Used to relieve menopause symptoms of all varieties.
K 3	Great Ravine	Go the highest point of the inner anklebone and slide backward halfway to the Achilles tendon.	Relieves symptoms of menopause, including mood swings, night sweats, and insomnia.
Sp 6	Three Yin Crossing	Three finger-widths above the inner anklebone along the back of the tibia.	Promotes general balance for all issues of female regulation.
CV 6	Lower Sea of Qi	In the depression three chon below the belly button in the midline of the body.	Generally uplifting, rejuvenates qi flow, and relieves general weakness.
CV 17	Upper Sea of Qi	Exact center of the breastbone, halfway between the top and bottom, and then drop slightly lower.	Relieves hot flashes and calms nervous anxiety.

The following acupressure routine can be effective in alleviating the symptoms of menopause:

1. **Breathe, stretch, and ground yourself as in the acupressure routines that appear earlier in this chapter.**

2. **Use the following points in the following pattern; use sustained pressure on points that feel too empty and alternating pressure on points that feel too full.**

   Work each point for 1 to 3 minutes.

   - Use a bilateral hold on GB 20.

   - Press LI 11 on one arm, and then on the other.

   - Press H 6 on one arm, and then on the other.

   - Use a bilateral approach for Lv 3, K 3, and Sp 6.

   - Hold CV 6 and CV 17 together.

3. **You can use individual points any time you need them — H 6 and LI 11 are particular favorites!**

Reflexology for Overall Women's Health

Several studies have shown reflexology to be beneficial in treating female-specific ailments, especially PMS and menstrual cramps. This is partly because reflexology helps balance the body's systems, including hormone levels — the fluctuation of which can lead to problems such as PMS and menstrual pain. Here's a reflexology routine that can be helpful in addressing a variety of women's concerns:

1. **Start by washing and drying your feet.**

2. **If you haven't already stretched and performed deep breathing exercises, do some deep belly breathing now.**

3. **Sit in a chair or on a bed and cross your leg so that you can hold your foot in your lap.**

4. **Roll your foot back and forth in your hand, loosening up any restrictions.**

   Use horizontal stripping to further open the zones of your foot.

5. **Locate the reflex zones for female reproductive organs (see the reflexology map in Figure 17-5).**

   These points are on the top of the foot and along the Achilles tendon next to the anklebones. You can use them for all female issues, but they're especially great for PMS, fertility, and pregnancy.

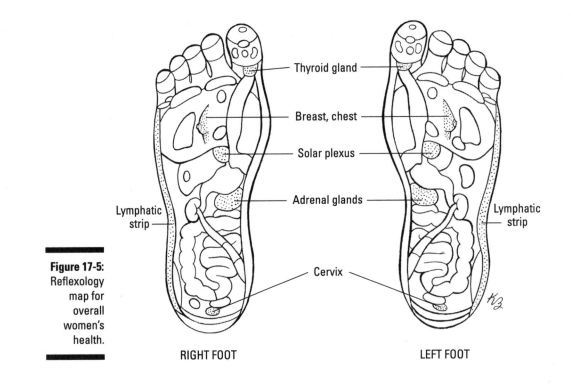

Thyroid gland

Breast, chest

Solar plexus

Adrenal glands

Lymphatic strip

Lymphatic strip

Cervix

Figure 17-5:
Reflexology map for overall women's health.

RIGHT FOOT   LEFT FOOT

6. **Massage and finger-walk these areas using circular motion on sore spots as needed.**

   Note: Be sure to avoid using pressure on the ankles — you might inadvertently stimulate Sp 6, which is a taboo point during pregnancy.

7. **On your reflexology map, find the reflex zones for the breasts, cervix, thyroid gland, and adrenal glands.**

   Thumb-walk these areas and use circular motion as needed.

8. **If you need them, find the reflex zones for breastfeeding stimulation, PMS symptoms, and/or menopause.**

   Thumb-walk these areas and use circular motion as needed.

9. **Use finger-walking along the lymphatic strip to help your body flush out toxins.**

   This step is especially important during pregnancy when you don't want toxins creating an imbalance in the system.

10. **End with thumb-walking and circular motions to the solar plexus and the adrenals to stimulate smooth qi flow.**

11. **Repeat with the other foot.**

12. **Relax, lie quietly, and breathe deeply, allowing qi flow to respond to the session.**

    You may notice warmth and tingling through your body as qi rebalances.

Chapter 18

Fighting Colds, Preventing Illness, and Relieving Some Chronic Conditions

Sure, everyone knows that major accidents and injuries can cause serious pain. But many people underestimate the impact that small maladies like the common cold, the flu, and other chronic conditions can have on your daily life.

Think about it: Are you really giving 100 percent at your job, at home, or anywhere else if you're distracted by those bothersome cold symptoms? Even minor symptoms like an annoying cough or a slight fever can prevent you from performing at your best. In addition, these pesky illnesses tend to linger and make themselves at home inside your body until they eventually wear you down and take a toll on your immune system and energy levels. That's why it's so important to nip these conditions in the bud, fighting them off before they grow into bigger problems.

By using acupressure and reflexology, you can keep these irritating cold and flu symptoms at bay. In addition, you can give your immune system the boost it needs to keep these nasty bugs from invading your space in the first place.

Boosting Your Immune System with Qi

The best way to deal with cold and flu symptoms is to avoid them altogether by keeping your immune system strong enough to fight off these germs before they ever get a chance to set up shop inside your body. Your immune system determines your ability to resist infection, degeneration, and the growth of abnormal cancerous cells. As we discuss in Chapter 1, according to Chinese medicine, your health and immune system depend on the proper balance and flow of qi. Qi nourishes and sustains the body; without balanced, harmonious, and adequate qi, you lose vital energy, which opens the door to illness.

By using bodywork to boost your immune system, you increase your resistance to illness of all kinds and have the greatest odds of avoiding these common maladies and more serious ailments. And if you're already feeling a little under the weather, acupressure can give your immune system the boost that it needs to fight off the invading illness. Familiarize yourself with the points in Table 18-1 if you want to know which points strengthen the immune system. If you want a visual reference, check out Figures 18-1, 18-2, and 18-3.

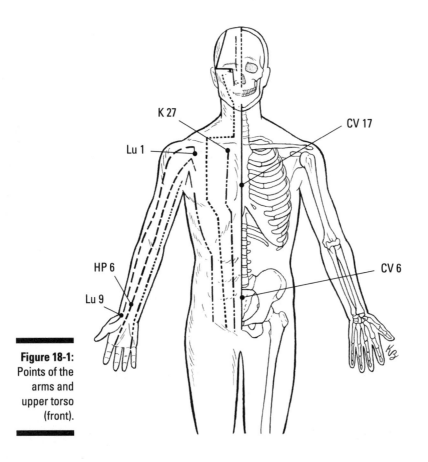

Figure 18-1:
Points of the
arms and
upper torso
(front).

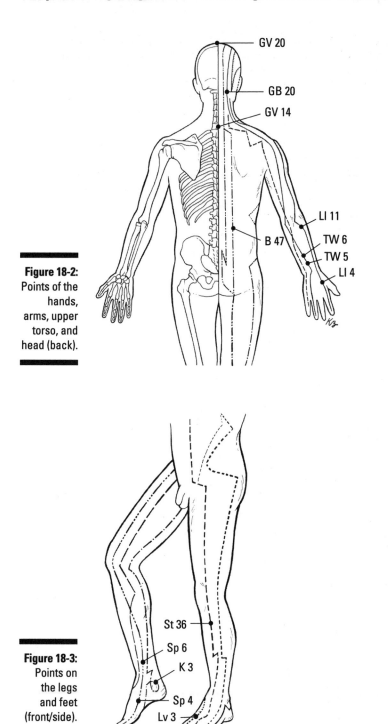

Figure 18-2:
Points of the
hands,
arms, upper
torso, and
head (back).

Figure 18-3:
Points on
the legs
and feet
(front/side).

Table 18-1		Points to Strengthen Immunity	
Point Abbreviation	**Name of Point**	**How You Find It**	**Benefits**
K 3	Great Ravine	Go the highest point of the inner anklebone and slide backward halfway to the Achilles tendon.	Strengthens the immune system.
Lv 3	Great Rushing	On the top side of the foot, go between the big and second toes; trace up the webbing between the metatarsal bones until the bones come together, forming a depression.	Boosts the immune system by invigorating the blood and regulating qi flow.
Sp 6*	Three Yin Crossing	Two chon (three finger-widths) above the inner anklebone along the back of the tibia.	Relieves immune weakness and restores vitality.
St 36	Three Mile Point	One chon out from the shinbone and three chon (one palm-width) below the patella.	Revitalizes body and immune functions.
K 27	Shu Mansion	Under the collarbone in the depression next to the breastbone.	Strengthens the immune system.
LI 11	Crooked Pond	At the top of the elbow crease, on the edge of the joint.	Relieves immune weakness.
CV 17	Upper Sea of Qi	Go to the center of the breastbone, halfway between the top and bottom, and move slightly down from the center.	Governs the body's resistance to illness by regulating the thymus gland. Also decreases anxiety.

* Never use this point during pregnancy.

The following routine is useful when you've been exposed to an illness or just want a little extra precaution:

1. **Belly breathe while centering and grounding (see Chapter 2).**

2. **Stretch your whole body to encourage qi flow to all areas by following these steps:**

   • Take your arms up over your head while breathing in and stretch backward as far as you comfortably can (don't overstretch and hurt yourself). Hold for the count of three.

   • Exhale as you bend forward, stretching your arms to the floor. Be a rag doll and hold this stretch for the count of three.

   • Inhale as you stand back up; bring your arms over your head and lean to the side, exhaling while you lean. Hold.

   • Breathe in as you straighten up and repeat the previous three steps on the other side.

   • Repeat the whole sequence three times to fully open the meridian channels.

3. **Work the points in Table 18-1, using sustained pressure on points that feel too empty or alternating pressure on points that feel too full.**

   Work each set of points for 1-3 minutes.

   • Use bilateral holds on K 3, Lv 3, and Sp 6. Press each one in turn and repeat until soreness is reduced or you have an overall sense of flow; repeat at least three times.

   • Use bilateral holds on St 36 and K 27. Alternate pressure between these two points for three rotations.

   • Alternately press LI 11 on both arms for approximately 3 minutes each. Repeat as necessary to reduce any soreness.

   • End by pressing CV 17 for 3 minutes.

4. **Follow with reflexology, or lie quietly and give yourself time to allow the qi to balance through your system.**

Ousting the Common Cold, Flu, and Fever

You may not think you can do much to cope with cold and flu symptoms, aside from taking some over-the-counter medication and waiting for the storm to pass. Well, you'll be pleasantly surprised to learn that acupressure can make a big difference in the effects of these common conditions. The immune system is comprised of white blood cells (WBC) that fight infection, cell destruction or degeneration, and cancer. With acupressure and reflexology, you can direct qi to stimulate WBC production and function, and you can direct it to areas that are weakened or under attack by infection.

Don't underestimate the seriousness of the flu. Each year, at least 30,000 deaths in the United States are attributed to the flu. Older people, babies, and people with health problems that leave their immune systems in a weakened state are most at risk.

Focusing on the points in Table 18-2 can help you survive this miserable experience. You can see these points in Figures 18-1 and 18-2, earlier in this chapter.

Table 18-2		Great Acupoints for Cold, Flu, and Fever	
Point Abbreviation	**Name of Point**	**How You Find It**	**Benefits**
LI 4*	Union Valley	In the webbing where the index finger and the thumb meet. If you close your finger and thumb, you'll find it at the bottom of the crease. You can pinch this point between your index finger and thumb.	Relieves congestion.
Lu 9	Great Abyss	On the palm side of the hand, under the thumb, in the wrist crease.	Regulates lung qi, resolves excess phlegm, and opens the chest.
TW 5	Outer Gate	Two chon (three finger-widths) above the wrist crease, on the outside of the forearm in the center between the two tendons.	Increases resistance to colds.
LI 11	Crooked Pond	At the top of the elbow crease, on the edge of the joint.	Relives cold symptoms and reduces fever.
GB 20	Wind Pool	Along the ridge of your occipital bone, halfway between your ear and spine, between the two muscles that come together.	Key point for relieving colds.

* Never use this point during pregnancy.

Use the following routine to encourage the white blood cells of your immune system to combat the viral, bacterial, or fungal invasion underway. If you don't have time to do all the points, choose the points that most match your symptoms. Press them with alternating pressure if they're too full or with sustained pressure if they're too empty.

1. **Belly breathe while centering and grounding.**

2. **Stretch the meridians in the arms and chest by following these steps:**

   • Stand with your feet shoulder-width — or farther — apart.

   • Slightly bend your knees.

   • Breathe in while raising your arms to shoulder level, palms down. Continue breathing in and spread your arms backward at shoulder-blade level while rotating your hands palms up. Reach your thumbs toward the floor behind you.

   • Exhale and relax, bringing your arms back to your side.

   • Repeat three times.

3. **Work the points in Table 18-2, using sustained pressure on points that feel too empty or alternating pressure on points that feel too full.**

   • Start with either arm and work LI 4, Lu 9, TW 5, and LI 11 for 1 to 3 minutes each. Repeat the series until all the points feel even.

   • Repeat on the other arm.

   • Use the bilateral approach on GB 20, alternating pressure on each point until they're even.

4. **Follow with reflexology or lie quietly and imagine your defense system actively destroying the microbes causing your illness.**

Flushing Out Toxins

One of the main causes of illness is toxic overload. Junk food, food additives, pollution, and toxic chemicals clog the system with harmful substances and interfere with cellular function. This can cause you to feel groggy, tired, and unmotivated with aches, pains, groans, and moans. Toxins decrease your body's defenses and contribute to degenerative conditions, such as arthritis. Repetitive or chronic illnesses are often indicative of toxic overload blocking the body's repair mechanisms.

Detoxification is an important step to acquiring better health and promoting a stronger immune system. The organs of detoxification and elimination of toxins are the liver, kidneys, colon, lungs, and skin. In the removal of stored toxins, these organs often take a toll. Be sure to drink plenty of water, six to eight 8-ounce glasses per day, to flush your system whenever you're initiating detoxification pathways.

Methods of detoxification include fasting or other dietary changes and/or herbs to initiate the cleansing process. Acupressure and reflexology can assist by sending qi to the organs involved. You can even use specific points to stimulate the removal of toxins and flush them from the system — check out Table 18-3 and refer to Figures 18-1, 18-2, and 18-3, earlier in this chapter.

Use both acupressure and reflexology together to promote detoxification, because each supports the other in this process.

Table 18-3		Detoxification with Acupressure	
Point Abbreviation	Name of Point	How You Find It	Benefits
Lv 3	Great Rushing	On the top side of the foot, go between the big and second toes; trace up the webbing between the metatarsal bones until the bones come together, forming a depression.	Regulates and tonifies the liver, a major detoxifying organ.
Sp 6*	Three Yin Crossing	Two chon (three finger-widths) above the inner anklebone along the back of the tibia.	Helps flush qi and blood through the body.
K 27	Shu Mansion	Under the collarbone in the depression next to the breastbone.	Tonifies the kidneys, another key detoxification organ.
LI 4*	Union Valley	In the webbing where the index finger and the thumb meet. If you close your finger and thumb, you'll find it at the bottom of the crease. You can pinch this point between your index finger and thumb.	Stimulates elimination and release of toxins through the bowels.
HP 6	Inner Gate	Palm side of the hand, in the middle of the arm, three finger-widths above the wrist crease between the two tendons.	Regulates stomach, heart, and liver qi.
CV 17	Upper Sea of Qi	Go to the center of the breastbone, halfway between the top and bottom, and move one chon down from the center.	Transforms qi and clears the chest, which houses the upper burner of the triple warmer meridian, allowing qi to flow freely through the lungs.
CV 6	Lower Sea of Qi	Three chon below the belly button on the midline of the body.	Relieves general fatigue and confusion and helps fortify the immune system.

Never use these points during pregnancy.

This routine helps clear your system of toxins and encourages a healthy immune system:

1. **Belly breathe while centering and grounding.**

2. **Stretch your whole body to encourage qi flow to all areas by following these steps:**

   - Take your arms up over your head while breathing in and stretch backward as far as you comfortably can (don't overstretch and hurt yourself). Hold for the count of three.

   - Exhale as you bend forward, stretching your arms to the floor. Be a rag doll and hold this stretch for the count of three.

   - Inhale as you stand back up; bring your arms over your head and lean to the side, exhaling while you lean. Hold for the count of three.

   - Breathe in as you straighten up and repeat the previous three steps on the other side.

   - Repeat the whole sequence three times to fully open the meridian channels.

3. **Work the points in Table 18-3, using sustained pressure on points that feel too empty or alternating pressure on points that feel too full.**

   Work each set of points for 1 to 3 minutes.

   - Use bilateral holds on Lv 3, Sp 6, and K 27. Repeat this sequence until the points feel even.

   - Start with either arm, and alternately hold LI 4 and HP 6. Repeat on the other arm. Continue until all four points are even and balanced.

   - Finish by holding CV 17 and CV 6 together for 1 to 3 minutes.

4. **Follow with reflexology or lie quietly, relaxing your muscles and allowing qi to flow easily and smoothly through your body.**

Combating Chronic Fatigue

Chronic fatigue is another long-term condition that leaves many people physically exhausted (hence the name). Often, it has no clear cause, which makes it difficult to treat. But many people have found bodywork techniques to be effective in alleviating the "always tired" feeling that this condition causes.

If your energy flow is blocked or disrupted, your endurance ability lags and you feel tired all the time (even when you first wake up in the morning). These symptoms can only add to the problems already faced by someone who suffers from chronic fatigue. By freeing your qi, you rev up your energy levels.

The routine in this section uses the points in Table 18-4, which are shown in Figures 18-1, 18-2, and 18-3, earlier in this chapter.

Table 18-4	Acupressure on Chronically Fatigued Points		
Point Abbreviation	Name of Point	How You Find It	Benefits
TW 4	Yang Pool	Go to the back of the hand to the wrist; find the point in the wrist crease, halfway between the inside and outside of the wrist, between the two tendons.	Regulates qi in the triple warmer meridian, and helps overall energy balance and flow.
K 27	Shu Mansion	Under the collarbone in the depression next to the breastbone.	Tonifies the kidneys, which manage and regulate the storage and release of qi.
St 36	Three Mile Point	One chon out from the shinbone and three chon below the patella.	Strengthens qi flow through the body.
Sp 4	Grandfather-Grandson	This point is on the medial side of the foot, one chon below the foot pad beneath the big toe. Find the bone in the arch of the foot, hook your finger into the arch from underneath, and press upward.	Rejuvenates the spleen meridian and nourishes the entire body.
B 62	Extending Vessel	On the outside of the foot, one and a half chon below the middle of the outer anklebone, in the indentation.	Used for chronic fatigue.
CV 6	Lower Sea of Qi	Three chon below the belly button on the midline of the body.	Relieves general fatigue and confusion.
GV 14	Great Hammer	At the big vertebrae where the neck meets the back.	Invigorates qi through the whole body, restores energy, calms the spirit, and clears the brain.

The following routine can help boost your energy levels, which can help you perform your daily routine more efficiently and just help you feel better overall.

1. **Belly breathe while centering and grounding.**

2. **Stretch your whole body to encourage qi flow to all areas by following these steps:**

   • Take your arms up over your head while breathing in and stretch backward as far as you comfortably can (don't overstretch and hurt yourself). Hold for the count of three.

   • Exhale as you bend forward, stretching your arms to the floor. Be a rag doll and hold this stretch for the count of three.

   • Inhale as you stand back up; bring your arms over your head and lean to the side, exhaling while you lean. Hold.

   • Breathe in as you straighten up and repeat the previous three steps on the other side.

   • Repeat the whole sequence three times to fully open the meridian channels.

3. **Work the points in Table 18-4, using sustained pressure on points that feel too empty or alternating pressure on points that feel too full.**

   Work each set of points for 1 to 3 minutes.

   • Start with either arm and hold TW 4, alternating arms until both points feel even.

   • Use bilateral holds on K 27, St 36, Sp 4, and B 62. Repeat the application of pressure on this set of points until the points feel balanced and even.

   • Hold CV 6 at the same time as GV 14 for 1 to 3 minutes.

4. **Follow with reflexology or relaxation.**

   During relaxation, your body and mind integrate the change of qi flow. You may notice a deeper state of relaxation than you normally feel with deeper breaths and fewer thoughts running around in your mind.

Immune Stimulation and Detox with Reflexology

Foot and hand reflexology is great to stimulate detoxification and build the immune system. The major organs for eliminating toxins are the kidneys, liver, lungs, large intestine, lymphatic system, and skin. You can stimulate each of these through the feet and hands, and most of them have specific reflex areas. In addition to supporting immune system function, detox is a great way to support weight loss and can help overcome the nasty side effects if you're quitting smoking.

The following reflexology routine can help boost your immune system while simultaneously helping your body get rid of harmful toxins:

1. **Start by washing and drying your feet.**

2. **If you haven't already stretched and performed deep-breathing exercises, do some deep belly breathing now.**

3. **Sit in a chair or on a bed and cross your leg so that you can hold your foot in your lap.**

4. **Use foot rolling and foot stripping to stretch the tissue, loosen restrictions, and open the reflex zones.**

   For directions, refer to Chapter 4.

5. **Thumb-walk, looking for any nodules, soreness, or crackling sounds, and then use circular motions to work out the tension.**

6. **Stimulate the reflex area to balance the adrenal glands (see Figure 18-4).**

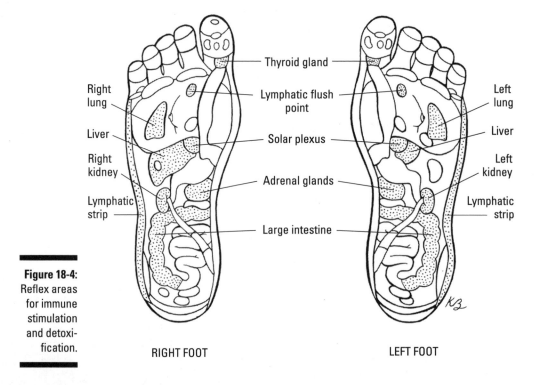

Figure 18-4: Reflex areas for immune stimulation and detoxification.

Thyroid gland

Right lung

Lymphatic flush point

Liver

Solar plexus

Right kidney

Adrenal glands

Lymphatic strip

Large intestine

Left lung

Liver

Left kidney

Lymphatic strip

RIGHT FOOT

LEFT FOOT

The adrenal glands, which regulate stress response, are just below the ball of the foot on the inside of the arch.

Adrenals are very helpful in regulating body processes that assist detoxification. In addition, overfunctioning of the adrenal glands produces too much *cortisol,* a stress hormone that inhibits the immune system. Balancing this reflex area can decrease stress, reduce cortisol production, and improve immune function.

7. **End with thumb-walking and circular motions to the solar plexus in the center of the foot, and the lymphatic strip on the outside edge of the foot.**

8. **Repeat with the other foot.**

9. **Relax to allow the body to fully adjust to the changes you have initiated.**

Part V
The Part of Tens

The 5th Wave   By Rich Tennant

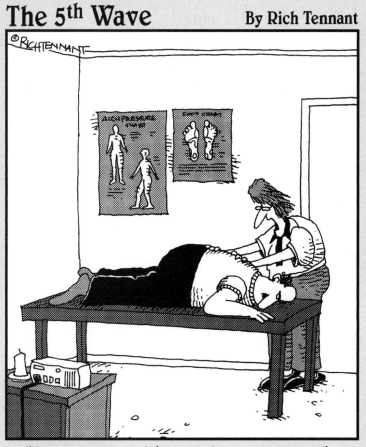

"I sense some tightness in your wallet."

In this part . . .

Part V is, of course, the Part of Tens. Our first segment tackles common myths and misconceptions of acupressure and reflexology. Chances are good that you've heard (and possibly even believed) at least one or two of these. Fortunately, we help you separate fact from fallacy. We continue on a positive note by spotlighting a few of the ways in which the healing arts can make a positive impact on your life.

Finally, we point you in the right direction for further information by including an appendix filled with resources where you can learn more about the topics of acupressure and reflexology. Whether you're curious about the history of the healing arts or just want further details on more specific topics related to bodywork, you'll find some helpful resources in this section.

Chapter 19

Ten Myths and Misconceptions About Acupressure and Reflexology

The healing arts of acupressure and reflexology are often misunderstood or incorrectly represented. In this chapter, we present some common fallacies surrounding these practices.

Acupressure Involves Needles

Different from acupuncture, acupressure involves no thin needles or sharp instruments at all (in fact, no instruments of any kind). Generally, the only "tools" involved are the practitioner's own two hands. Both acupuncture and acupressure, however, are guided by the principles of Chinese medicine, use acupoints to effect change in meridians, and employ a holistic approach to healing that includes mind, body, emotions, and spirit.

Acupressure and Reflexology Are Crazy, Short-Lived Fads

A lot of people believe that acupressure and reflexology are nothing more than a crazy fad. This belief couldn't be further from the truth. In reality, acupressure and reflexology both have their roots in ancient Chinese medicine. People of various cultures have been practicing them for thousands of years.

So, in comparison to the ancient roots of acupressure and reflexology, you may say that many of the newer popular healing treatment methods used today — such as many modern cutting-edge techniques — are really short-lived fads.

The Healing Arts Are Connected to Black Magic and Other Spiritual Stuff

Perhaps you're reluctant to try acupressure and reflexology because you heard that they're tied to black magic. This is totally false — acupressure and reflexology have no connection to black magic or anything scary at all. A basic tenet of the healing arts is the importance and power of positive thoughts and good energy. The healing arts have been (and continue to be) employed by people of all walks of life and many different religions. This belief originated because the concept of energy is so foreign. In general, people are afraid of what they don't know. Science does not yet have the equipment to measure qi directly (skin measurements are indirect measurements of skin conductivity, not direct measurements of an energy output), and research on the effects and benefits of acupuncture, acupressure, and other energy medicine has been scanty. As such, it has easily been misunderstood. Fortunately this is all changing. Medical research is now more plentiful, and the benefits of energy modalities are more accepted.

Healing Requires Special Powers or Complicated Training

Not true. Healing doesn't require any special powers or complicated training. Everyone has the power to heal. You just need to embrace your abilities and have confidence in your own innate ability to heal. True, specialized training is essential for the more complicated, in-depth, professional use of acupressure and reflexology. However, a few simple guidelines are all you need for the basic techniques and simple applications presented in this book.

Healing Techniques Require Lots of Time

Healing techniques don't necessarily take a lot of time. You can devote as much or as little time as you're willing and/or able to spare. Obviously, the more time you can devote to healing, the better results you can often achieve. The routines in this book can easily be applied in 20 to 30 minutes;

however, when you have a headache, foot problem, or so on, spending just 5 minutes pressing the appropriate points can make a big difference in how you feel, and in your energy levels.

The Healing Arts Are a Substitute for Conventional Care

The healing arts definitely aren't a substitute for conventional care, and we want to stress that emphatically. The healing arts are used in conjunction with (and as a complement to) necessary medical treatment, not as a replacement. No ethical and responsible healing-arts practitioner would ever claim that these techniques can cure cancer, diabetes, MS, or any other serious medical condition. You should always seek a doctor's care for any painful or chronic medical condition, or for a serious accident, illness, or injury. However, bodywork *can* stimulate the body's healing mechanism and relieve some of the pain and other symptoms that are caused by these and other medical conditions.

The Healing Arts Are Dangerous for Certain People

The assumption that the healing arts are dangerous for certain groups of people is false, for the most part. In general, acupressure and reflexology are completely safe for almost everyone. It is true, however, that youngsters, pregnant women, and others may need adjustments to general sessions. Session time may need to be reduced, and specific movements or certain points may need to be avoided. In this book we alert you to such adjustments as needed. Also, people who are extremely delicate or weak should, of course, use caution (and perhaps consult their doctor) before embarking on any kind of healing routine.

Acupressure and Reflexology Techniques Are Painful

Some people believe that acupressure and reflexology techniques are painful. False. On the contrary, these techniques should make you feel at least a little bit better, often immediately. In some cases, you may experience what's sometimes called "good pain," similar to what you may feel with a really deep stretch or a good massage. However, you should never experience any actual pain — and if you do, you should stop immediately. After a session, some people may experience a *healing crisis,* which is an exacerbation of symptoms prior to resolution.

Acupressure and Reflexology Are Fancy Names for Garden-Variety Massages

Massage is certainly one of the healing arts, and acupressure and reflexology do involve some basic massage techniques, but they aren't the same as your garden-variety massage. Massage, acupressure, and reflexology all employ detailed, specific approaches based on scientific foundations involving the roots of pain and basic physiology. They all have a holistic approach to wellness, interacting with mind, body, and spirit. However, acupressure and reflexology are much more complex practices that include assessing and balancing the flow of energy along meridian or reflex pathways.

Energy Is Transferable

Many people believe that one person's energy is transferred to another in healing practices. We can't speak for all healing practices, but acupressure and reflexology don't exchange energy between giver and receiver. A basic assumption of this work is that the receiver has everything he needs within himself; it's just out of balance or harmony. Acupressure and reflexology seek to balance the energy of the receiver, not give the receiver energy or take it away.

Chapter 20

Ten Ways Acupressure and Reflexology Can Enrich Your Life

In This Chapter

▶ Helping you feel better

▶ Improving your relationships with others

Acupressure and reflexology can have many positive effects on your life — physically, emotionally, and mentally. In this chapter, we address a few of the major benefits you can enjoy by taking part in bodywork sessions.

You're More Relaxed

Perhaps the most immediately obvious benefit of bodywork sessions is that you're more relaxed. From practically the moment a session starts, you most likely begin to feel increasingly relaxed. And when practiced regularly, bodywork leaves you more relaxed in general.

Acupressure and reflexology both encourage deep tranquility and relaxation by restoring the optimal flow of energy throughout your body, helping your body release the negative energy brought on by stress. By promoting the proper flow of qi and helping to remove any energy blockages, which can be stressful, bodywork allows you to enjoy a more relaxed state no matter what you may be doing. See Chapters 1 and 3 to learn more about the importance of proper qi flow.

You Lessen the Effects of Stress

Bodywork treatments can also help alleviate the physical symptoms of stress, such as increased muscle tension, which can cause headaches, stiffness, and muscle pain; elevated blood pressure, which contributes to heart disease; or feelings of anxiety brought on by feeling stressed out. Relieving physical symptoms of stress can put your body in a better energetic state to handle whatever stressful situations you can't avoid.

Your Life is More Balanced

A basic principle of both acupressure and reflexology is the restoration of harmonious energy flow, putting qi in proper balance. In Chinese medicine, all illness and distress in life can be attributed to imbalances of qi. So balancing qi brings you more balance and stability, physically, mentally, and emotionally. As a result, you enjoy better health, a more positive attitude, fewer aches and pains, and better decision-making skills. In short, a more balanced life overall!

You're More in Tune with Your Body

Acupressure and reflexology both encourage you to become more aware of your body. This heightened awareness makes you much more sensitive to your body's natural rhythms and its optimum state. When you have this heightened awareness, you're often able to immediately notice any deviation from your body's optimum state or any disruption to your energy flow. As a result, you can sometimes nip problems in the bud, treating an energy blockage while it's still in an early state, before it grows into a more disruptive condition.

Another added benefit of becoming more aware of your body: You have a greater appreciation for all the amazing and wonderful things your body does on a daily basis. You may be surprised to discover just how many things you had taken for granted!

You're in Less Pain

Acupressure and reflexology almost always lessen pain. Obviously, if you've suffered a severe injury or if you're dealing with a debilitating disease, bodywork treatments can do only so much. However, for routine pains caused by minor to moderate injuries, illnesses, and other conditions, the healing arts are often very effective in reducing your pain and making you more comfortable.

You Enjoy Better Relationships

Enjoying better relationships with those around you does tend to happen, for a variety of reasons. First, face it — people who are in pain tend to be a bit crabby. If you feel better physically, you also have a better outlook on life and are probably a much more pleasant person to be around. People are drawn to you and enjoy being in your company. Also, when your energy flow is in sync and you have emotional balance, you tend to enjoy more positive relationships with loved ones and interact better with professional colleagues.

You Have More Energy

Acupressure and reflexology are both focused on restoring a person's proper balance and flow of qi. As a result, your energy is no longer blocked or slowed down, and you're able to enjoy more of this positive fuel. Also, people who are uncomfortable or in pain tend to feel less motivated and less energetic. By alleviating some of your pain, bodywork techniques can in turn leave you feeling more invigorated and optimistic about life in general. Pressure point therapies, as well as massage and other bodywork techniques, have the added benefit of increasing the release of endorphins. *Endorphins* are neurotransmitters released in nerve synapses that stimulate feelings of well-being, relaxation, and inner calm. This combination of beneficial effects provides you with the optimum combination of more energy, greater alertness, and clam relaxation. Bottom line: You feel ready to go out and conquer the day!

You Heal Faster

One of the main goals of acupressure and reflexology is to encourage and accelerate the healing process by stimulating the proper flow of energy to the correct parts of the body. This helps your body heal itself naturally. The body is designed with self-healing mechanisms that require proper fuel and conditions to work. Physiologically, every cell needs nutrients, removal of waste products, fuel from the food you eat, oxygen, and water. In Chinese medicine, vitality, supplied by qi, is included in that list. All physical substances are supplied to cells by the circulatory system, so when circulation is diminished, cell health is compromised. The principle demonstrated through acupressure and reflexology is that where qi goes, blood follows. When the channels of qi are open, cells receive vitality and circulation is improved, providing the cells with all they need to heal faster.

In addition, acupressure and reflexology also encourage emotional well-being, and this positive state often helps speed up the healing and recovery process. Many studies have demonstrated a connection between positive thinking and faster healing. For example, a study published in the July 2006 issue of the *Journal of the American Academy of Orthopedic Surgeons* showed that refraining from stress, worry, and other negative emotions played an important role in speeding patients' recovery.

You Have More Self-Confidence

By performing these techniques on yourself and others, you start to discover the fact that you have the power to heal yourself. This discovery can be emotionally and mentally empowering, and can really give your self-confidence a big boost.

You Nurture Yourself

If you're like most people, you spend lots of time taking care of everyone else, and very little time taking care of yourself. Most likely, you often neglect your own physical and emotional needs — even when you're in pain.

Engaging in acupressure and reflexology sessions forces you to treat yourself to some "me time," which you most likely desperately need. This "me time" is far from selfish — the better you feel, the more efficiently you can fulfill all your daily duties and nurture the important people in your life.

Appendix

Resources

● ●

Many acupressure and reflexology resources can help you to further your skills and understanding. After you get started, you may find that you want more and more!

Web Sites

There are many online sites that cover various aspects of bodywork and healing arts. Here are a few that we think you'll find helpful:

✔ www.holisticlink.net: This site gives you a good description of different types of alternative healthcare, including acupressure and reflexology. It also provides book reviews and lists and has links to professional organizations and schools.

✔ www.naturalhealers.com: Check out this comprehensive education resource for people pursuing careers in the natural healing arts. It provides information on licensure, training requirements, certification programs, job growth, salaries, and more.

✔ www.yinyanghouse.com: This is a great Web site for Traditional Chinese Medicine. It has a section for acupressure that includes books for animal acupressure, self-acupressure, and practitioner treatment. It also has practitioner listings to help you find a therapist in your area.

✔ www.naturalhealthweb.com: This site is a good resource for articles and information on alternative health methods.

Professional Organizations

Bodywork associations have been getting more organized in the face of changing state regulations. Associations offer a wide variety of services. They're often involved in legally helping to define the field and creating state and national standards of practice and training. You can log on to the associations' Web sites to find a licensed or certified therapist near you; to find a list of certified schools and resources; to obtain professional liability insurance; or to find out the legal requirements in your state for becoming a professional. These sites can also provide information on continuing education, new book critiques, and sales of books and tools:

- ✔ **American Oriental Body Therapies Association (AOBTA):** This organization's Web site (www.aobta.org) is the most comprehensive association for acupressure with the largest membership base.

- ✔ **American Massage Therapy Association (AMTA):** The AMTA Web site (www.amtamassage.org) can direct you to massage schools where you can find reflexology and acupressure programs.

- ✔ **The American Reflexology Certification Board (ARCB):** This is an association of reflexologists working to set national certification standards. Its Web site (www.arcb.net) can direct you to training centers and practitioners.

- ✔ **National Certification Board for Therapeutic Massage and Bodywork (NCBTMB):** The NCBTMB provides certification standards for the fields of massage and bodywork, establishing agreed-upon codes of ethics and standards of practice. It establishes and administers the National Certification Exam used in all state licensing for massage therapists, which may include reflexology or acupressure. Its Web site tells you about state licensing requirements and exam procedures, has member profiles, and lists certificants who have violated the nationally established codes of ethics or standards of practice. The organization also receives complaints from receivers.

Training Centers

Innumerable bodywork training centers around the country offer certification in acupressure and/or reflexology. Many states require a massage therapy license in order to practice acupressure, so many massage therapy schools offer secondary certification programs in acupressure and/or reflexology. Other massage schools offer a few classes as adjunctive therapies, which is fine if acupressure or reflexology isn't your primary interest. The following schools and training centers offer high-quality programs that meet professional standards.

Acupressure training

If you're thinking that you may like to pursue further acupressure education (perhaps to practice professionally), here are some places where you can obtain training.

Acupressure Therapy Institute

This school offers a 720-hour, approved training program in an eclectic shiatsu acupressure program. Shiatsu is one type of the original forms of acupressure practiced in Japan. It's the best-known method, and we have incorporated many shiatsu practices in this book, including finger pressure techniques and stretching.

For more information, contact

Barbara Blanchard, Director and President
1 Billings Road
Quincy, MA 02171
Phone 617-697-1477
Fax 617-253-2156
E-mail info@acupressuretherapy.com
Web site www.acupressuretherapy.com

CenterPoint Massage & Shiatsu Therapy School & Clinic

This school teaches two complete and different systems of shiatsu: Namikoshi Shiatsu and Shiatsu Amma. Learning these styles offers the practitioner a versatile and expansive vocabulary in shiatsu therapy.

For more information, contact

Cari Johnson Pelava, Director
1313 5th Street SE #336
Minneapolis, MN 55414
Phone 612-617-9090
Fax 612-617-9292
E-mail info@centerpointmn.com
Web site www.CenterPointMN.com

The Jin Shin Do Foundation for Bodymind Acupressure

This school offers training in emotional and mind-body aspects of acupressure. The program meets national accreditation standards and has the advantage of offering intensive weeklong courses of study at various locations internationally. This is an ideal program for those who aren't near a fixed location school or can't schedule the traditional semester approach to learning.

For more information, contact

Iona Marsaa Teeguarden, Director
P.O. Box 416
Idyllwild, CA 92549
Phone 951-659-5707
Fax 951-659-5707
E-mail teegers@earthlink.net
Web site www.JinShinDo.org

Ohashi Institute

The Ohashi Institute was founded in 1974 and established the form of acupressure known as Ohashiatsu. Using more than just traditional philosophy and meridian balancing, Ohashiatsu focuses on communication and synergy between giver and receiver, including development of the physical, psychological, and spiritual harmony of both.

For more information, contact

Wataru Ohashi, Director
147 West 25th Street, 6th Floor
New York, NY 10001
Phone 800-810-4190
E-mail info@ohashiatsu.org

Pacific College of Oriental Medicine

Pacific College of Oriental Medicine was founded in 1986. It provides oriental medical and body therapy education to students from around the world. Campuses exist in San Diego, New York, and Chicago, where a student can learn acupuncture, acupressure, oriental herbs, and other aspects of oriental medicine.

For more information, contact

Jack Miller, President
7445 Mission Valley Road, Suite 105
San Diego, CA 92108
Phone 800-729-0941
Fax 619-574-6641
E-mail admissions-sd@PacificCollege.edu
Web site www.PacificCollege.edu

Zen Shiatsu Chicago

Zen Shiatsu was established by Shizuto Masunaga (1925–1981), a Japanese psychologist who was born into a family of shiatsu practitioners but decided to create his own new form of the art. His approach emphasizes the meditative connection between the practitioner and client. The practice seeks to balance the yin and yang forces in the body.

For more information, contact

Steve Rogne, Director
825A Chicago Avenue
Evanston, IL 60202
Phone 847-864-1130
Fax 847-864-1131
E-mail info@zenshiatsuechicago.org
Web site www.zenshiatsuchicago.org

Reflexology training

Reflexology is taught in massage schools and through certified programs offered around the country. Reflexology has many forms, and most stem from the Ingham Method developed in the early 1900s. One of the most popular alternatives is the Universal Method, which was developed in the 1980s.

- ✔ **International Institute of Reflexology, Inc.:** This is the home of the Ingham Method of reflexology, which is the oldest form of reflexology being practiced in the United States today. It's considered the basic modern technique from which most others are derived. Check out the Web site at www.reflexology-usa.net.

- ✔ **Connecticut Center for Universal Reflexology:** The Universal Method was developed in South Africa by Chris Stormer, who founded the Reflexology Academy of Southern Africa in 1989. It's a gentler form of reflexology that has gained international popularity. Find out more at www.universalreflexology.net.

- ✔ **International Institute of Advanced Reflexology:** Founded in 1989, this organization was formed with the goal of raising the practice of reflexology to the highest professional level. Licensed by the Pennsylvania State Board of Private Licensed Schools and the U.S. Department of Education. Web site: www.reflexology.net.

- ✔ **American Academy of Reflexology:** A nationally accredited school devoted exclusively to reflexology, the Academy offers classes for beginners, as well as continuing education for professional practitioners. Web site: www.americanacademyofreflexology.com.

- ✔ **Academy of Ancient Reflexology:** The Academy's professional certification program blends traditional Eastern philosophies with modern Western approaches. Web site: www.academyofancientreflexology.com.

Books

We tried to make this book as informative as possible, but bodywork is a vast topic that encompasses lots of issues and ideas. Here are some books that can provide you with more insight into specific topics related to the healing arts.

Philosophy of Chinese medicine

If you enjoy reading about the basic ideas and philosophy of Chinese medicine in Chapter 1, you may want to check out these two books. They're considered to be classics in the field. They're clear and easy to read (sort of), so you shouldn't feel too overwhelmed by new and different thinking.

✔ *The Web That Has No Weaver,* by Ted J. Kaptchuk (McGraw-Hill)

✔ *Between Heaven and Earth,* by Harriet Beinfield and Efrem Korngold (Ballantine Books)

Body-mind medicine

Does the information in Chapter 7 on your body, mind, and emotions fascinate you? Body-mind medicine has become one of the fastest-growing areas of interest. Here are three great resources for more information:

✔ *Molecules of Emotion,* by Candace B. Pert (Simon & Schuster): This book is filled with original scientific research that establishes the physiology of the body-mind connection. It's readable, easy to understand, and fascinating!

✔ *Bodymind,* by Ken Dychtwald (Tarcher Putnam): This book explains how tension in the body is related to emotions and explores the areas in which emotions are felt and expressed. It's engaging and easy to read.

✔ *The Joy of Feeling,* by Iona Marsaa Teeguarden (Japan Publications): This book makes the connection between emotions, areas of the body, and meridians. It provides acupoints and simple treatments for emotional health. A little more studious, it covers case studies and offers a wealth of practical information.

Acupressure practice

If you enjoy doing acupressure, you may want more instruction. Books are a great resource, but you'll find many different approaches to acupressure. Don't get confused! Here are some books that offer clear, simple, and easy-to-use instruction in several of the main types of acupressure. You may want to see which form of acupressure fits you best.

✔ *Acupressure Way of Health: Jin Shin Do,* by Iona Marsaa Teeguarden (Japan Publications): This book is the best guide for the layperson into the magic of body-mind based acupressure. An absolute must for those looking to explore deeper patterns of health and healing.

✔ *Amma Therapy,* by Tina Sohn and Robert Sohn (Healing Arts Press): Amma is a complex system of bodywork that incorporates massage and acupoints. It dates back 5,000 years. This book combines the ancient practice with modern approaches and includes nutrition and exercise recommendations to help balance meridians.

✔ *Beyond Shiatsu,* by Wataru Ohashi and Ken Okano (Kodansha America): This book is a comprehensive guide to the Ohashi method of acupressure that incorporates traditional and modern approaches. This method stresses an interaction between practitioner and receiver that's uplifting, beneficial, and growth-oriented for both. A gentle and effective form of acupressure.

✔ *The Complete Book of Shiatsu Therapy,* by Toru Namikoshi (Japan Publications): A compact yet comprehensive and scientifically oriented guidebook to restore self-healing powers. This book uses medical science, traditional philosophy, and informative technique to guide the reader to shiatsu practice.

✔ *The Complete Guide to Acupressure: Jin Shin Do,* by Iona Marsaa Teeguarden (Japan Publications): This book offers a comprehensive approach to explaining the many facets of Chinese medicine and theory with practical, insightful instruction. The Jin Shin Do Bodymind Acupressure technique focuses on the body, mind, and emotional aspects of acupressure.

✔ *Shiatsu: The Complete Guide,* by Chris Jarmey, Gabriel Mojay, and Peter Cox (Thorsons Publishers): This book includes easy-to-follow instructions on classic shiatsu technique.

✔ *Zen Shiatsu,* by Shizuto Masunaga, Wataru Ohashi, and the Shiatsu Education Center of America (Japan Publications): A spiritually based shiatsu practice that relies on analysis of yin/yang balance and the five-element theory to asses and restore health. Zen shiatsu is a technique that seeks to develop inner resources in both practitioner and client.

Reflexology practice

Here are two good books on two main reflexology methods, the Ingham Method and the Universal Method:

✔ *Better Health with Foot Reflexology,* by Dwight C. Byers (Ingham Publishing, Inc.): Fully explains this method in easy-to-understand language with plenty of charts and instruction.

✔ *Language of The Feet,* by Chris Stormer (Hodder & Stoughton): Chris Stormer pioneered the Universal Method of Reflexology. This is her first book and it clearly explains her approach and gives down-to-earth, practical information.

And here are a couple other reflexology books that you may enjoy:

✔ *The Busy Person's Guide to Reflexology,* by Ann Gillanders (Barron's Educational Series): A short book designed to be a quick read, this provides simple basic routines designed to be performed in 5 minutes or less.

✔ *Clinical Reflexology,* by Peter Mackereth (Churchill Livingstone): A technical book designed for professionals (or aspiring professionals), this book covers the theory and practice of reflexology.

Index

• *Q* •

BUSINESS, CAREERS & PERSONAL FINANCE

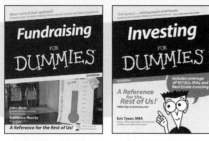

0-7645-9847-3

0-7645-2431-3

Also available:
- Business Plans Kit For Dummies
  0-7645-9794-9
- Economics For Dummies
  0-7645-5726-2
- Grant Writing For Dummies
  0-7645-8416-2
- Home Buying For Dummies
  0-7645-5331-3
- Managing For Dummies
  0-7645-1771-6
- Marketing For Dummies
  0-7645-5600-2
- Personal Finance For Dummies
  0-7645-2590-5*
- Resumes For Dummies
  0-7645-5471-9
- Selling For Dummies
  0-7645-5363-1
- Six Sigma For Dummies
  0-7645-6798-5
- Small Business Kit For Dummies
  0-7645-5984-2
- Starting an eBay Business For Dummies
  0-7645-6924-4
- Your Dream Career For Dummies
  0-7645-9795-7

HOME & BUSINESS COMPUTER BASICS

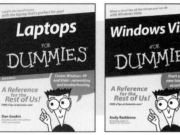
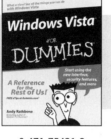

0-470-05432-8

0-471-75421-8

Also available:
- Cleaning Windows Vista For Dummies
  0-471-78293-9
- Excel 2007 For Dummies
  0-470-03737-7
- Mac OS X Tiger For Dummies
  0-7645-7675-5
- MacBook For Dummies
  0-470-04859-X
- Macs For Dummies
  0-470-04849-2
- Office 2007 For Dummies
  0-470-00923-3
- Outlook 2007 For Dummies
  0-470-03830-6
- PCs For Dummies
  0-7645-8958-X
- Salesforce.com For Dummies
  0-470-04893-X
- Upgrading & Fixing Laptops For Dummies
  0-7645-8959-8
- Word 2007 For Dummies
  0-470-03658-3
- Quicken 2007 For Dummies
  0-470-04600-7

FOOD, HOME, GARDEN, HOBBIES, MUSIC & PETS

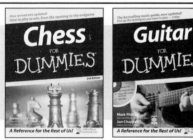

0-7645-8404-9

0-7645-9904-6

Also available:
- Candy Making For Dummies
  0-7645-9734-5
- Card Games For Dummies
  0-7645-9910-0
- Crocheting For Dummies
  0-7645-4151-X
- Dog Training For Dummies
  0-7645-8418-9
- Healthy Carb Cookbook For Dummies
  0-7645-8476-6
- Home Maintenance For Dummies
  0-7645-5215-5
- Horses For Dummies
  0-7645-9797-3
- Jewelry Making & Beading For Dummies
  0-7645-2571-9
- Orchids For Dummies
  0-7645-6759-4
- Puppies For Dummies
  0-7645-5255-4
- Rock Guitar For Dummies
  0-7645-5356-9
- Sewing For Dummies
  0-7645-6847-7
- Singing For Dummies
  0-7645-2475-5

INTERNET & DIGITAL MEDIA

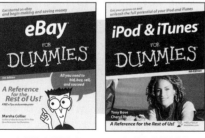

0-470-04529-9

0-470-04894-8

Also available:
- Blogging For Dummies
  0-471-77084-1
- Digital Photography For Dummies
  0-7645-9802-3
- Digital Photography All-in-One Desk Reference For Dummies
  0-470-03743-1
- Digital SLR Cameras and Photography For Dummies
  0-7645-9803-1
- eBay Business All-in-One Desk Reference For Dummies
  0-7645-8438-3
- HDTV For Dummies
  0-470-09673-X
- Home Entertainment PCs For Dummies
  0-470-05523-5
- MySpace For Dummies
  0-470-09529-6
- Search Engine Optimization For Dummies
  0-471-97998-8
- Skype For Dummies
  0-470-04891-3
- The Internet For Dummies
  0-7645-8996-2
- Wiring Your Digital Home For Dummies
  0-471-91830-X

* Separate Canadian edition also available
† Separate U.K. edition also available

Available wherever books are sold. For more information or to order direct: U.S. customers visit www.dummies.com or call 1-877-762-2974.
U.K. customers visit www.wileyeurope.com or call 0800 243407. Canadian customers visit www.wiley.ca or call 1-800-567-4797.

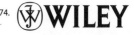

SPORTS, FITNESS, PARENTING, RELIGION & SPIRITUALITY

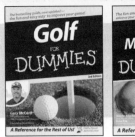

0-471-76871-5

0-7645-7841-3

Also available:
- Catholicism For Dummies
  0-7645-5391-7
- Exercise Balls For Dummies
  0-7645-5623-1
- Fitness For Dummies
  0-7645-7851-0
- Football For Dummies
  0-7645-3936-1
- Judaism For Dummies
  0-7645-5299-6
- Potty Training For Dummies
  0-7645-5417-4
- Buddhism For Dummies
  0-7645-5359-3

- Pregnancy For Dummies
  0-7645-4483-7 †
- Ten Minute Tone-Ups For Dummies
  0-7645-7207-5
- NASCAR For Dummies
  0-7645-7681-X
- Religion For Dummies
  0-7645-5264-3
- Soccer For Dummies
  0-7645-5229-5
- Women in the Bible For Dummies
  0-7645-8475-8

TRAVEL

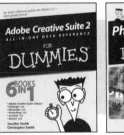

0-7645-7749-2

0-7645-6945-7

Also available:
- Alaska For Dummies
  0-7645-7746-8
- Cruise Vacations For Dummies
  0-7645-6941-4
- England For Dummies
  0-7645-4276-1
- Europe For Dummies
  0-7645-7529-5
- Germany For Dummies
  0-7645-7823-5
- Hawaii For Dummies
  0-7645-7402-7

- Italy For Dummies
  0-7645-7386-1
- Las Vegas For Dummies
  0-7645-7382-9
- London For Dummies
  0-7645-4277-X
- Paris For Dummies
  0-7645-7630-5
- RV Vacations For Dummies
  0-7645-4442-X
- Walt Disney World & Orlando
  For Dummies
  0-7645-9660-8

GRAPHICS, DESIGN & WEB DEVELOPMENT

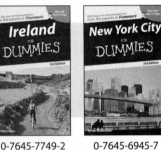

0-7645-8815-X

0-7645-9571-7

Also available:
- 3D Game Animation For Dummies
  0-7645-8789-7
- AutoCAD 2006 For Dummies
  0-7645-8925-3
- Building a Web Site For Dummies
  0-7645-7144-3
- Creating Web Pages For Dummies
  0-470-08030-2
- Creating Web Pages All-in-One Desk
  Reference For Dummies
  0-7645-4345-8
- Dreamweaver 8 For Dummies
  0-7645-9649-7

- InDesign CS2 For Dummies
  0-7645-9572-5
- Macromedia Flash 8 For Dummies
  0-7645-9691-8
- Photoshop CS2 and Digital
  Photography For Dummies
  0-7645-9580-6
- Photoshop Elements 4 For Dummies
  0-471-77483-9
- Syndicating Web Sites with RSS Feeds
  For Dummies
  0-7645-8848-6
- Yahoo! SiteBuilder For Dummies
  0-7645-9800-7

NETWORKING, SECURITY, PROGRAMMING & DATABASES

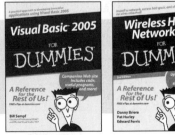

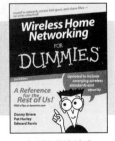

0-7645-7728-X

0-471-74940-0

Also available:
- Access 2007 For Dummies
  0-470-04612-0
- ASP.NET 2 For Dummies
  0-7645-7907-X
- C# 2005 For Dummies
  0-7645-9704-3
- Hacking For Dummies
  0-470-05235-X
- Hacking Wireless Networks
  For Dummies
  0-7645-9730-2
- Java For Dummies
  0-470-08716-1

- Microsoft SQL Server 2005 For Dummies
  0-7645-7755-7
- Networking All-in-One Desk Reference
  For Dummies
  0-7645-9939-9
- Preventing Identity Theft For Dummies
  0-7645-7336-5
- Telecom For Dummies
  0-471-77085-X
- Visual Studio 2005 All-in-One Desk
  Reference For Dummies
  0-7645-9775-2
- XML For Dummies
  0-7645-8845-1

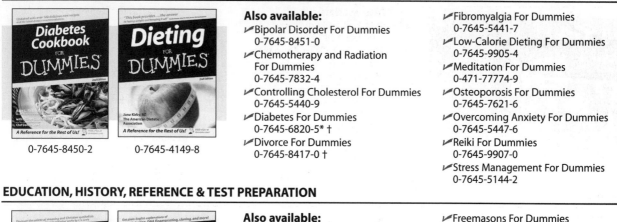
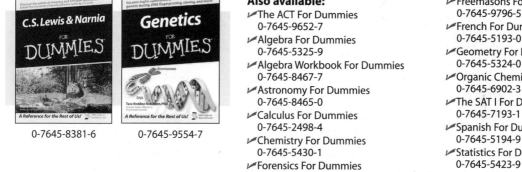
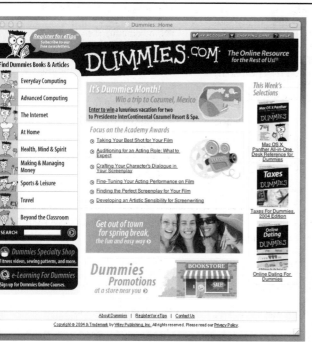
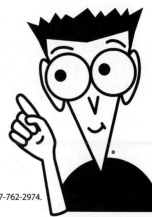

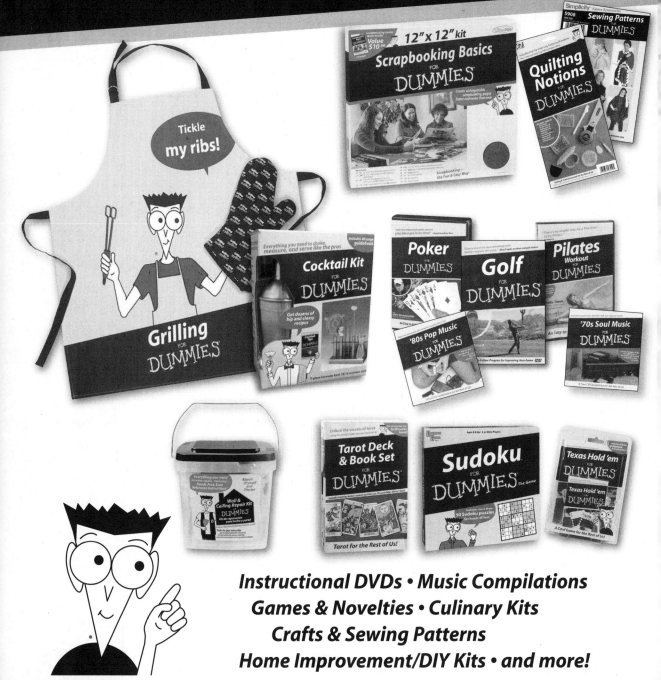
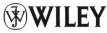